PREGNANCY DIET COOKBOOK FOR FIRST TIME MOMS

The Flavorful Journey: Explore Delicious Choices to keep you energized and support your baby's development

Dr. Angela C. Williams

TABLE OF CONTENTS

CONCLUSION

INTRODUCTION

Welcome to The Pregnancy Diet Cookbook – a practical guide born out of a journey that began with a simple yet profound realization. As a soon-to-be mother myself, I found navigating the world of pregnancy nutrition overwhelming. There was a flood of information, contradictory advice, and the constant worry about providing the best for my unborn child. In the midst of this confusion, a pivotal moment emerged that not only eased my worries but inspired the creation of this cookbook.

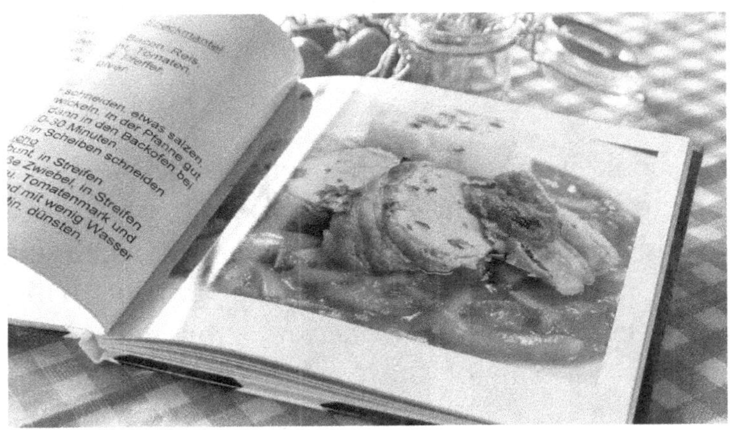

During my own pregnancy, I stumbled upon a treasure trove of wisdom from experienced mothers and nutrition experts. It wasn't about fancy diets or complicated theories; it was about practical, real-life experiences and simple yet effective recipes that kept both mother and baby healthy. This collection of insights became the foundation of The Pregnancy Diet Cookbook, and I am thrilled to share it with you.

One particular story stands out in my memory. A group of expectant mothers, facing similar dilemmas, gathered to share their experiences and learn from each other. In those conversations, we discovered the power of nourishing our bodies with the right foods. The transformations were remarkable – not just physically, but emotionally and mentally as well. It was this shared journey that sparked the idea for a cookbook that goes beyond recipes, offering a holistic approach to pregnancy nutrition.

This book is not about imposing strict rules or advocating for complex dietary plans. Instead, it's a friendly companion, simplifying the overwhelming task of nourishing yourself and your growing baby. Each recipe is crafted with care, grounded in the collective wisdom of those who have walked this path before.

As you embark on this journey with me, I invite you to embrace the simplicity within these pages. No need for elaborate culinary skills or exotic ingredients – just a willingness to prioritize your well-being and your baby's health. Together, let's discover the joy of nurturing life through mindful and enjoyable eating.

So, whether you are a first-time mom or a seasoned parent, let The Pregnancy Diet Cookbook be your guide, providing not only nourishing recipes but also a source of comfort and support. As we delve into the pages ahead, remember that your journey is unique, and this book is here to empower you to make choices that resonate with your individual needs.

Now, turn the page and let the adventure begin. To a healthy and fulfilling pregnancy journey await you. The power to shape this remarkable experience is in your hands.

Take the first step towards a vibrant and nourished pregnancy. Your story starts here.

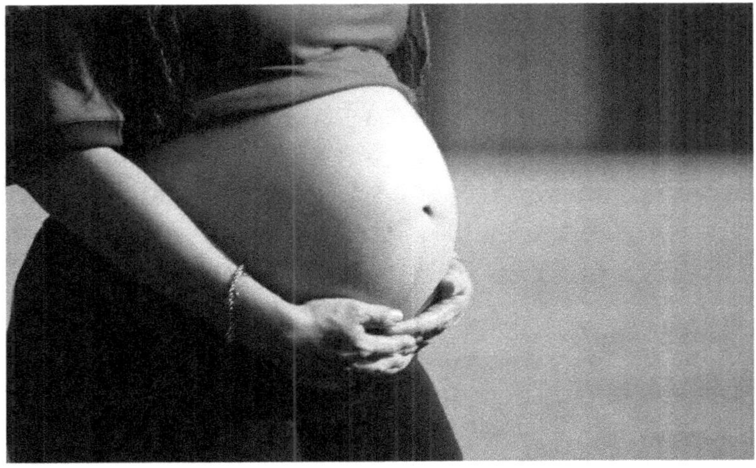

NOURISHING BEGINNINGS - THE IMPORTANCE OF A HEALTHY PREGNANCY DIET

In the quiet whispers of life's most profound moments, the miracle of creating life emerges. One such moment, the journey through pregnancy, is a tapestry woven with the threads of anticipation, joy, and responsibility. As I embark on sharing the wisdom gathered from my own journey, let us explore the cornerstone of a healthy pregnancy - a well-balanced and nutritious diet.

A Personal Prelude

Before delving into the science, let me take you back to a quiet afternoon when the reality of impending parenthood set in. Cradling a positive pregnancy test in my hands, the magnitude of responsibility suddenly felt tangible. Excitement mingled with a hint of trepidation. That evening, as the sunset cast a warm glow on our home, my partner and I vowed to provide the best possible start for our little one.

Understanding the Significance

The journey of pregnancy is akin to nurturing a delicate seed into a vibrant blossom. The role of nutrition in this journey cannot be overstated. Imagine a garden where each nutrient is a caretaker, ensuring the soil is rich, the water pure, and the sunlight ample. Similarly, a healthy pregnancy diet lays the foundation for the optimal development of the tiny life growing within.

Nutrients: The Building Blocks

Consider the nutrients as the architects of your baby's development. Folic acid, for instance, plays a crucial role in preventing neural tube defects. It's like a skilled craftsman, intricately shaping the foundation of the nervous system. Iron becomes the sturdy pillars, supporting the oxygen transport to your baby, fostering growth and vitality.

A Symphony of Taste and Health

*Contrary to the myth that a healthy pregnancy diet is a bland affair, let me assure you, it's a culinary symphony. Picture a plate adorned with a vibrant array of colors – greens, reds, yellows. These colors signify a diverse range of fruits and vegetables, each contributing essential vitamins and minerals. It's not just about eating for one; it's about indulging in a gastronomic celebration for two.

Empowering Choices

Our journey led us to a profound realization – the power of choices. Just as an artist selects the finest brush for a masterpiece, an expectant mother crafts her baby's health through mindful food choices. Opting for whole grains, lean proteins, and healthy fats is like selecting the finest materials to build a strong and resilient foundation.

A Dance of Hydration

In the tapestry of pregnancy, hydration is the silent choreographer. Water, the unsung hero, orchestrates the dance of nutrients, ensuring a seamless flow to the baby's growing abode. It's like the refreshing rain, quenching the thirst of both the earth and the seeds it nurtures.

The Emotional Tapestry

Pregnancy is not just a physical journey but an emotional one. The food we consume shapes not only the baby's physical development but also their emotional well-being. Imagine each nutrient as a tender embrace, nurturing the baby's emotional fabric.

Navigating Cravings and Aversions

The enigmatic cravings and aversions – my personal companions on this journey. While the sudden longing for pickles might seem whimsical, it often carries a hidden message. Our bodies, in their infinite wisdom, signal the need for specific nutrients. Listening to these cues is like decoding the secret language of pregnancy.

The Ripple Effect

As we embraced this journey, the positive effects of a healthy pregnancy diet rippled through our lives. Increased energy levels, better mood, and a sense of empowerment became our constant companions. The benefits extended beyond the confines of pregnancy, leaving an indelible mark on our overall well-being.

Cultivating a Supportive Environment

Just as a garden thrives in a nurturing environment, so does a growing life within. Surrounding oneself with a supportive network – be it a partner, family, or healthcare professionals – ensures that the journey is not a solitary one. Sharing the joys, challenges, and questions creates a collective wisdom that propels you forward.

Conclusion: A Nourished Tomorrow

In the gentle rhythm of the baby's first kicks, the heartbeats on the monitor, and the whispers of lullabies, the essence of a healthy pregnancy diet reveals itself. It's a journey of love, care, and commitment to providing the best possible start for the newest member of the family.

As I reflect on my personal voyage, I can't help but marvel at the transformative power of nourishment. A healthy pregnancy diet is not a prescription but a love letter to the life blossoming within. It's an investment in a future where health, vitality, and joy intertwine to create a tapestry that spans generations.

May your journey be as vibrant and fulfilling as the colors on your plate. Here's to nourishing beginnings and the symphony of life that unfolds with each carefully chosen bite.

NUTRITIONAL GUIDELINES FOR EXPECTING MOTHERS

Congratulations on this incredible journey into motherhood! As you embark on the beautiful path of pregnancy, it's crucial to prioritize your health and nutrition. Ensuring you get the right nutrients not only benefits you but also plays a vital role in the development of your little one. Let's dive into some straightforward and practical nutritional guidelines for expecting mothers.

1. Balanced Diet - The Foundation

The cornerstone of a healthy pregnancy is a balanced diet. Aim to include a variety of foods from different food groups in your meals. This means a good mix of:

a. Fruits and Vegetables:

- Load up on colorful fruits and veggies to get a range of vitamins and minerals.
- Opt for dark, leafy greens like spinach and kale for added iron and folic acid.

b. Whole Grains:

- Choose whole grains like brown rice, quinoa, and whole wheat bread for fiber and essential nutrients.

c. Protein Sources:

- Include lean proteins like poultry, fish, beans, and tofu for muscle development and overall growth.

d. Dairy or Alternatives:

- Ensure you're getting enough calcium for bone development. Milk, yogurt, and fortified plant-based milk are good options.

e. Healthy Fats:

- Avocado, nuts, and olive oil provide essential fatty acids crucial for the baby's brain and nervous system.

2. Folic Acid - A Pregnancy Superhero

Folic acid is a superhero nutrient during pregnancy. It helps prevent neural tube defects in the baby's brain and spine. Ensure you're getting enough by incorporating:

- Leafy greens
- Fortified cereals
- Legumes
- Oranges and orange juice

Your healthcare provider may also recommend a folic acid supplement, so discuss this with them.

3. Iron - The Oxygen Carrier

Iron is essential for both you and your baby's health. It helps carry oxygen to your cells and prevents anemia. Iron-rich foods include:

- Lean meats
- Beans and lentils
- Fortified cereals
- Spinach and broccoli

Pair iron-rich foods with vitamin C sources (like citrus fruits) to enhance absorption.

4. Calcium - Strong Bones Ahead

Calcium is crucial for the development of your baby's bones and teeth. Include these calcium-rich options in your diet:

- Dairy products (milk, cheese, yogurt)
- Fortified plant-based milk
- Leafy greens (like kale and bok choy)

5. Hydration - The Unsung Hero

Staying hydrated is often overlooked but is vital during pregnancy. Water helps form the amniotic fluid, carries nutrients to your baby, and prevents constipation. Aim for at least 8-10 glasses of water daily.

6. Small, Frequent Meals - The Pregnancy Hack

Instead of three large meals, opt for smaller, more frequent meals. This can help manage nausea, heartburn, and keep your energy levels stable throughout the day.

7. Limit Caffeine and Sugar Intake

While a cup of coffee is okay, excessive caffeine intake is best avoided during pregnancy. Too much sugar can lead to unnecessary weight gain. Opt for natural sweeteners and limit your intake of sugary snacks and beverages.

8. Safe Seafood Choices

Fish is an excellent source of omega-3 fatty acids, important for your baby's brain development. However, some fish may contain high levels of mercury, which can harm the baby's nervous system. Choose low-mercury options like salmon, shrimp, and tilapia.

9. Watch for Food Safety

Pregnant women are more susceptible to foodborne illnesses. Ensure that your food is properly cooked, and avoid raw or undercooked eggs, meats, and seafood. Also, steer clear of unpasteurized dairy products and soft cheeses.

10. Listen to Your Body

Lastly, pay attention to your body's signals. If you're craving a certain food, indulge in moderation. If a particular food makes you feel unwell, it's okay to avoid it. Trust your instincts and communicate any concerns with your healthcare provider.

Conclusion

Remember, you're not just eating for one; you're nourishing a growing life within you. By following these nutritional guidelines and maintaining open communication with your healthcare provider, you're providing the best possible start for your baby. Embrace this journey, savor each moment, and relish the joy of nurturing life within you. Here's to a healthy and happy pregnancy!

CHAPTER 1:
BUILDING A STRONG FOUNDATION

Welcome to the journey of building a strong foundation for a fulfilling and purpose-driven life. Just like constructing a sturdy house requires a solid base, so does creating a life that stands resilient in the face of challenges and blossoms with success. Let's embark on this exploration together, weaving personal experiences into the fabric of wisdom and practical insights.

The Blueprint of Life

Think of your life as a grand architectural project. You are the architect, and every decision you make is like laying a brick in the construction of your existence. It all begins with a blueprint – a vision for the life you want to build.

Personal Experience:
For me, this journey started with a simple question: What kind of life do I want to lead? This introspective moment became my blueprint, guiding me through the twists and turns of life.

1. Define Your Core Values

The foundation of any solid structure lies in its core values. These are the principles that define who you are and guide your choices.Think for a moment about what is most important to you. Is it honesty, kindness, or maybe resilience? Your core values act as a compass, steering you in the right direction when faced with life's crossroads.

Personal Experience:
My core value of integrity became my north star. It led me through tough decisions, ensuring that my actions aligned with my beliefs, even when the path seemed challenging.

2. Cultivate a Growth Mindset

Just as a building needs to adapt to different weather conditions, so do you in the ever-changing landscape of life. Embrace a growth mindset – the belief that your abilities and intelligence can be developed through dedication and hard work. Challenges become opportunities for growth, and setbacks are mere detours on the road to success.

Personal Experience:
Encountering setbacks in my career, I chose to see them as stepping stones rather than roadblocks. This

mindset shift allowed me to bounce back stronger and more resilient.

3. Invest in Education and Skill Development

Education is the cornerstone of personal development. Whether through formal education or continuous self-learning, acquiring knowledge is like reinforcing the walls of your life's structure. Equip yourself with skills that not only match your passions but also align with the demands of the ever-evolving world.

Personal Experience:
Investing time and effort in learning new skills not only broadened my horizons but also opened doors to opportunities I hadn't imagined.

4. Build Healthy Relationships

Imagine your life as a community within the larger city of humanity. Strong, supportive relationships are like the pillars that hold up your structure. Be in the company of positive and inspiring individuals. Cultivate meaningful connections that contribute positively to your growth.

Personal Experience:
Navigating through personal challenges, the support of friends and family became my anchor. Their

encouragement fueled my determination to keep building, even when the storm clouds gathered.

5. Prioritize Physical and Mental Well-being

A robust structure requires regular maintenance. Your physical and mental well-being is the maintenance crew for your life. Exercise, proper nutrition, and mindfulness practices are the tools that keep your structure standing tall against the tests of time.

Personal Experience:
In moments of stress, prioritizing self-care became my secret weapon. A rejuvenated mind and body allowed me to face challenges with newfound strength.

6. Embrace Failure as a Stepping Stone

No construction project is without hiccups. Similarly, failures are inevitable in the journey of life. Rather than viewing them as roadblocks, see them as opportunities to learn, grow, and refine your foundation. Every setback serves as a springboard for achievement.

Personal Experience:
Facing a business venture failure, I realized it was not the end but a redirection. Learning from that experience, I pivoted towards a more fulfilling path.

Conclusion: Laying the First Bricks

As we conclude this chapter, envision your life as a work in progress. Every decision, every experience, and every relationship adds a layer to your foundation. By defining your values, fostering a growth mindset, investing in education, building meaningful relationships, prioritizing well-being, and embracing failure, you are not just constructing a life; you are crafting a masterpiece.

Personal Experience:
Through the journey of building my own foundation, I discovered the joy of shaping my destiny. With each brick laid, I found fulfillment in the process, not just the destination. So, take pride in every step of this construction, for you are the architect of your extraordinary life. Let's turn the next page and continue this fascinating journey together.

ESSENTIAL NUTRIENTS FOR PREGNANCY

Welcome to the heart of your pregnancy journey, where we unravel the mysteries of essential nutrients crucial for both your well-being and the flourishing life growing within you. As we delve into this chapter, I'll share insights from my own journey, weaving personal experiences into the tapestry of nutritional wisdom.

Folic Acid: The Guardian of Neural Tube Development

Imagine folic acid as the vigilant guardian overseeing the construction of your baby's neural tube — the delicate structure that forms the spine and brain. During the early weeks of my pregnancy, I marveled at the significance of this nutrient. Leafy greens, fortified cereals, and beans became my allies, as I ensured a daily intake to provide a robust foundation for my baby's developing nervous system.

But why the emphasis on folic acid? Well, my friends, it's the superhero nutrient that significantly reduces the risk of neural tube defects. This protective role dawned on me as I felt the first flutter of kicks, realizing that each movement was a testament to the intricate dance of development orchestrated by the nutrients I diligently incorporated into my diet.

Iron: The Mighty Blood Support

As I ventured into the second trimester, the focus shifted to iron – the mighty supporter of blood production. I vividly recall moments of fatigue that sent me searching for iron-rich foods like lean meats, spinach, and beans. Iron became the unsung hero fueling the increased blood volume needed to nurture both my own body and the tiny being flourishing within.

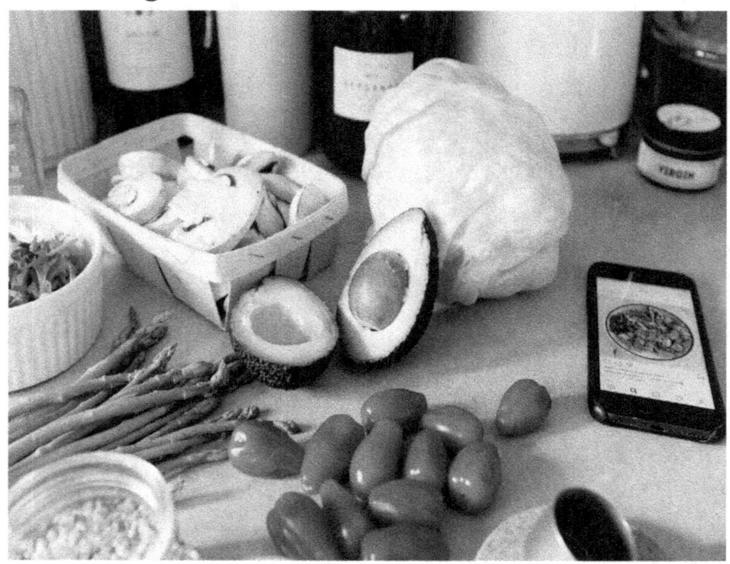

Let's not forget the pairing strategy – introducing vitamin C-rich foods to enhance iron absorption. It was like orchestrating a symphony of flavors on my plate, creating meals that not only satisfied my taste buds but also nurtured my body in its increased demand for this vital nutrient.

Calcium: The Architect of Strong Bones and Teeth

As my pregnancy progressed, calcium took center stage, emerging as the architect of my baby's developing bones and teeth. Dairy products, fortified plant-based milk, and leafy greens became foundational elements in my diet. And yes, being a vegetarian, I navigated the terrain of fortified alternatives, discovering a myriad of options to ensure my calcium intake remained robust.

Reflecting on this phase, I understood that calcium wasn't just a nutrient; it was a silent supporter, laying the groundwork for the skeletal structure that would soon cradle the essence of my motherhood.

Omega-3 Fatty Acids: Nourishing the Brain and Beyond

Omega-3 fatty acids, particularly DHA, took the spotlight as I entered the third trimester. These remarkable nutrients played a crucial role in nurturing my baby's developing brain and eyes.

Fatty fish, chia seeds, and walnuts became frequent visitors to my plate, contributing to the intricate tapestry of my baby's neurological foundation.

However, being cautious about mercury levels in certain fish became part of my dietary navigation. It was a learning curve, a reminder that while omega-3s were vital, making informed choices was equally important for the safety of my growing bundle of joy.

Protein: The Builders of Cells and Tissues

Proteins, the builders of cells and tissues, emerged as indispensable players throughout my pregnancy journey. Lean meats, poultry, fish, eggs, legumes, and nuts became the diverse cast in the nutritional drama unfolding within me. The realization struck – each protein-packed bite was contributing to the intricate cellular ballet propelling my baby's growth.

Incorporating proteins wasn't merely a dietary checklist; it was an acknowledgment of the dynamic role they played in shaping the physical foundation of my baby. It was a reminder that the act of nourishing went beyond satisfying cravings; it was a deliberate effort to provide the raw materials for life's extraordinary creation.

Vitamins and Minerals: The Unsung Heroes of the Ensemble

Beyond the spotlight nutrients, a symphony of vitamins and minerals played their unique tunes in the background of my pregnancy. Vitamin D, sourced from sunlight and fortified foods, danced alongside vitamin C, found in vibrant fruits and vegetables, facilitating iron absorption.

Minerals like zinc, magnesium, and iodine joined the ensemble, each contributing to the nuanced choreography of my baby's development. It was a holistic approach, a recognition that nutritional harmony relied on the collective efforts of these unsung heroes.

In Conclusion: Nurturing Life, One Nutrient at a Time

As I reflect on the journey through essential nutrients, I am reminded of the profound connection between the food I consumed and the intricate ballet of life unfolding within me. Each nutrient, each choice, resonated beyond a mere dietary decision – it was an investment in the vitality and well-being of both myself and my unborn child.

In embracing the essence of this chapter, I encourage you to recognize the significance of these essential nutrients. Picture them as the artisans crafting the masterpiece of your pregnancy, infusing life with each carefully chosen meal. As you navigate this nutritional odyssey, may the wisdom shared here guide you in nurturing life, one nutrient at a time.

Here's to the remarkable journey of motherhood, sculpted by the artistry of essential nutrients.

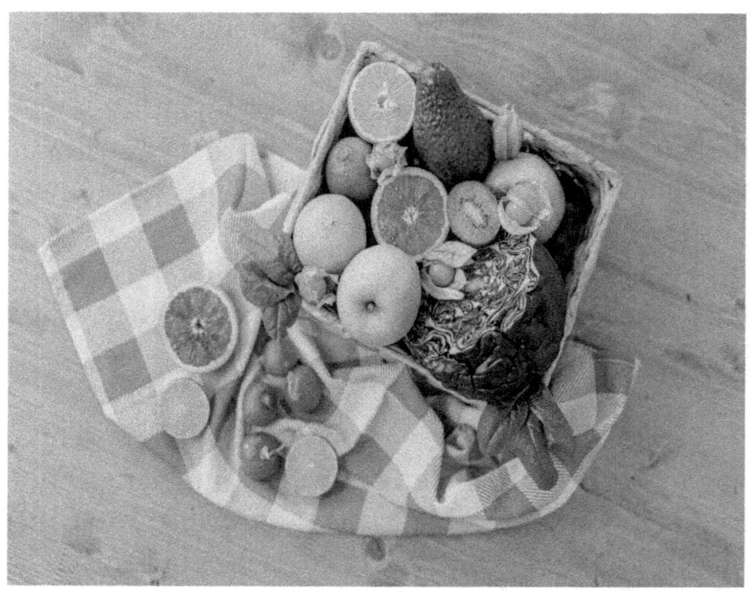

CREATING A BALANCED PLATE

Eating a balanced diet isn't just a health fad; it's a simple and effective way to ensure your body gets the nutrients it needs to function optimally. One key to achieving this is by creating a balanced plate with a variety of foods that provide essential vitamins and minerals. Let's break down the components of a balanced plate and explore some practical tips to help you achieve a well-rounded and nutritious meal.

The Foundation: Half Your Plate with Colorful Vegetables

The cornerstone of a balanced plate is an abundance of colorful vegetables. Vegetables are abundant in antioxidants, fiber, vitamins, and minerals. Aim to fill half of your plate with a variety of vegetables, including leafy greens, bell peppers, carrots, broccoli, and more.

Practical Tip 1: Mix it Up
Rotate your vegetable choices to ensure a diverse range of nutrients. Different colors often indicate various nutrients, so having a mix of colors ensures you get a broad spectrum of health benefits.

Practical Tip 2: Try Different Cooking Methods
Experiment with cooking methods such as roasting, steaming, or sautéing to keep things interesting. This can also bring out different flavors in your vegetables.

The Supporting Cast: Lean Proteins and Whole Grains

Now that you have a colorful veggie base, let's add some protein and whole grains. Proteins are crucial for muscle repair and growth, while whole grains provide sustained energy and essential nutrients.

Practical Tip 3: Choose Lean Proteins
Opt for lean protein sources like chicken, turkey, fish, tofu, or legumes. These choices are lower in saturated fats and provide essential amino acids your body needs.

Practical Tip 4: Embrace Whole Grains
Add healthful grains such as whole-wheat pasta, quinoa, or brown rice. Whole grains offer more fiber and nutrients compared to refined grains, promoting better digestion and sustained energy levels.

The Finishing Touch: Healthy Fats and Dairy (or Alternatives)

Healthy fats and dairy or dairy alternatives can complement your balanced plate by providing essential nutrients like omega-3 fatty acids and calcium.

Practical Tip 5: Choose Healthy Fats
Incorporate foods like avocados, almonds, seeds, and olive oil that are good sources of fat. These fats support heart health and can help you feel more satisfied after a meal.

Practical Tip 6: Opt for Low-Fat Dairy or Alternatives
If you include dairy, choose low-fat or fat-free options. Alternatively, explore dairy alternatives like almond milk or soy milk for those who are lactose intolerant or prefer plant-based options.

Mindful Eating: Portion Control and Hydration

Creating a balanced plate isn't just about the types of foods; it's also about portion control and staying hydrated.

Practical Tip 7: Practice Portion Control
Be mindful of portion sizes to avoid overeating. Use smaller plates to help control portions and prevent loading up more than your body needs.

Practical Tip 8: Stay Hydrated
Don't forget about hydration! Water is essential for overall health. Aim to drink an adequate amount of water throughout the day, and consider water-rich foods like fruits and vegetables.

Putting it All Together: Sample Balanced Plate Ideas

Now, let's put these practical tips into action with some sample balanced plate ideas:

Plate 1: Grilled Chicken Salad Plate
- Half the plate: Mixed greens, cherry tomatoes, cucumber slices
- Quarter of the plate: Grilled chicken breast
- Quarter of the plate: Quinoa or brown rice
- Finish with a drizzle of olive oil for healthy fats.

Plate 2: Vegetarian Stir-Fry Plate
- Half the plate: Stir-fried broccoli, bell peppers, snap peas
- Quarter of the plate: Tofu or chickpeas for protein
- Quarter of the plate: Brown rice or whole-grain noodles
- Add sliced avocado for healthy fats.

In Conclusion

Creating a balanced plate is a simple yet effective way to support your overall health and well-being. By incorporating a variety of colorful vegetables, lean proteins, whole grains, healthy fats, and hydration, you can ensure that your body receives the nutrients it needs to thrive. Remember, it's not about perfection but making small, sustainable changes that contribute to a healthier lifestyle. So, the next time you prepare a meal, think about the balance on your plate, and savor the goodness that comes with it.

THE ROLE OF HYDRATION IN A HEALTHY PREGNANCY

Water – the unsung hero of a healthy pregnancy. In this chapter, we'll dive into the vital role hydration plays in nurturing both you and your growing baby. From quenching your thirst to supporting critical bodily functions, let's explore the practical tips for maintaining optimal hydration throughout this extraordinary journey.

Understanding the Significance:

Hydration isn't just about satisfying your thirst; it's a cornerstone of a healthy pregnancy. Water is the vehicle that transports nutrients to your baby, helps maintain amniotic fluid levels, and supports the increase in blood volume your body needs. Think of it as the lifeblood flowing through the veins of your pregnancy.

Practical Tips for Hydration:

1. Keep a Water Buddy:
   Make friends with a water bottle – carry it with you everywhere. Having a water buddy by your side serves as a constant reminder to sip regularly.

Consider investing in a reusable bottle for an eco-friendly approach.

2. Set Hydration Reminders:

Pregnancy can be a whirlwind, and sometimes, hydration takes a backseat. Set hourly reminders on your phone or use apps designed to nudge you to drink water regularly. It's a simple yet effective way to stay on top of your hydration game.

3. Infuse Your Water:

If plain water feels mundane, infuse it with a burst of flavor. Add slices of cucumber, a hint of mint, or a splash of citrus for a refreshing twist. Experiment with different combinations to find your signature infused water.

4. Snack on Hydrating Foods:

Hydration isn't solely about liquids; some foods carry a high water content. Watermelon, cucumber, celery, and oranges are hydrating snacks that contribute to your daily fluid intake. Snack time becomes a dual-purpose delight!

Hydration and Common Pregnancy Symptoms:

Hydration plays a strategic role in addressing common pregnancy discomforts.

1. Morning Sickness:
   Sipping on ginger tea or ice-cold water can help alleviate nausea. Experiment with different temperatures to discover what feels soothing for you. The goal is to stay hydrated while providing comfort.

2. Constipation:
   Adequate water intake is a gentle remedy for constipation. It keeps things moving in your digestive system, promoting regular bowel movements. Remember, fiber and water work hand in hand for digestive harmony.

3. Preventing Swelling:
   Swelling, a common pregnancy woe, can be managed with hydration. Counterintuitive as it may seem, drinking more water helps your body release excess fluids, reducing swelling in ankles and feet.

Personal Insight:

During my pregnancy, staying hydrated became a personal ritual. I adorned my water bottle with encouraging stickers, turning it into a visual affirmation of nourishment. Infusing water with a slice of lemon became a daily act of self-care, a moment to pause and prioritize my well-being.

The Emotional Connection to Hydration:

Hydration is not just a physical practice; it's an emotional connection to your baby's well-being. Picture each sip as a gesture of love, nurturing, and dedication to the beautiful life growing within you. It's a silent conversation, a promise to provide the best possible environment for your little one.

In Conclusion: Sip, Nourish, Thrive:

As you traverse the landscape of pregnancy, let hydration be your constant companion. Sip, nourish, and thrive – it's a simple yet profound mantra. In every drop of water, envision the vitality it brings to both you and your baby.

Here's to the rhythmic flow of hydration, a symphony of well-being echoing through the corridors of your pregnancy journey.

CHAPTER 2
FIRST TRIMESTER : SETTING THE STAGE

The first trimester is like the overture to a symphony – setting the stage for the grand performance ahead. However, it comes with its own set of challenges, particularly the infamous morning sickness. Here are some practical tips:

1. Small, Frequent Meals: Instead of three large meals, consider smaller, more frequent ones. This can help manage nausea and keep your energy levels stable.

2. Folic Acid Focus: The early weeks are crucial for fetal development. Ensure a good intake of folic acid through foods like leafy greens, fortified cereals, and legumes.

3. Hydration Matters: Sip water throughout the day to stay hydrated. Dehydration can worsen nausea, so keep a water bottle handy.

NAUSEA AND MORNING SICKNESS :
A MORNING SYMPHONY

Morning sickness – the overture to many pregnancies. In the early days, my mornings felt like a delicate symphony, and the last thing I wanted was a discordant note of nausea. Here are some harmonious food choices:

1. Ginger Infusions: Ginger, whether in tea or as ginger ale, became my soothing melody. Its anti-nausea properties can help settle your stomach. Keep ginger candies or ginger-infused water on hand for a quick, natural remedy.

2. Simple Carbohydrates: Plain crackers, rice cakes, or toast played the role of the calming background melody. These easy-to-digest, simple carbohydrates can ease the queasiness.

3. Refreshing Citrus: Citrus fruits like lemons and oranges brought a zesty tune to my mornings. Sipping on water with a splash of lemon or indulging in citrusy snacks provided a refreshing relief from nausea.

Heartburn: Taming the Fiery Dragon

As the pregnancy journey progressed, heartburn entered the scene – a fiery dragon disrupting the gastronomic harmony. But fear not, for there are food choices that can help douse the flames:

1. Low-Acid Fruits: Opt for fruits with lower acidity, such as bananas, melons, and pears. These fruity companions can satisfy your sweet cravings without stoking the heartburn fire.

2. Lean Proteins: Lean meats, poultry, and fish became the knights in shining armor. These protein choices were not only gentle on my stomach but also aided in maintaining a feeling of fullness, reducing the likelihood of heartburn.

3. Whole Grains: Embrace the wholesome nature of whole grains like brown rice, quinoa, and oats. They are gentle on the stomach and provide sustained energy, helping to keep heartburn at bay.

Constipation: A Gentle Ballet of Fiber and Hydration

Constipation – the subtle ballet of discomfort. As my pregnancy journey advanced, I found a delicate dance between fiber-rich foods and hydration to be the perfect choreography:

1. Fiber-Rich Fruits: Prunes, apples, and berries gracefully entered the scene. These fiber-rich fruits contributed to the gentle rhythm of digestion, promoting regular bowel movements.

2. Leafy Greens and Vegetables: The verdant partners – spinach, kale, and broccoli – offered not only a symphony of nutrients but also acted as gentle agents in promoting healthy digestion.

3. Hydration Elegance:Water, the unsung hero, played a pivotal role. Maintaining soft stools requires being hydrated. Infusing water with slices of cucumber or a hint of mint added a touch of elegance to my hydration routine.

Balancing Cravings and Nutritional Needs: A Flavorful Waltz

Cravings, those unpredictable dance partners, added a unique flavor to my pregnancy journey. Balancing them with nutritional needs became a flavorful waltz:

1. **Sweet Cravings**: Instead of succumbing to refined sugars, I opted for nature's sweetness – fresh fruits, yogurt with a drizzle of honey, or a homemade smoothie became my delectable alternatives.

2. **Salty Cravings**: Nuts, seeds, and whole-grain crackers became the salty dancers in my craving waltz. They satisfied the salt cravings while contributing essential nutrients.

3. **Protein-Packed Indulgences**: Craving something indulgent? Chocolate protein balls or nut butter on whole-grain toast provided a satisfying compromise, offering a blend of pleasure and nutrition.

In Conclusion: A Symphony of Supportive Foods

Navigating pregnancy symptoms is akin to conducting a symphony – each section requiring its own melody. As you explore smart food choices, remember that this is your unique composition. Listen to your body, embrace the rhythms of each symptom, and allow food to be your supporting orchestra.

Through the ups and downs of nausea, heartburn, constipation, and cravings, let the food choices be the soothing notes in your symphony. May your pregnancy journey be harmonious, flavorful, and filled with the nourishment both you and your baby deserve.

Here's to a symphony of supportive foods guiding you through the beautiful crescendo of pregnancy symptoms.

BREAKFAST BOOSTERS :
ENERGIZING YOUR MORNINGS

Mornings during pregnancy can be a delicate dance between fatigue and the promise of a new day. In this chapter, I'll share breakfast boosters that not only energized my mornings but also set the tone for a day filled with vitality and nourishment. Join me in exploring simple yet powerful additions to your breakfast routine, enhancing both flavor and well-being.

1. Power-Packed Smoothies: A Sip of Vitality

Personal Insight: Mornings were a bit of a challenge for me during pregnancy, and the idea of a heavy breakfast was often unappealing. Enter the power-packed smoothie – a game-changer. Blending fruits, greens, and protein transformed my mornings into a vibrant symphony of flavors and energy.

Ingredients for a Berry Green Smoothie:
- One cup of mixed berries, comprising raspberries, blueberries, and strawberries
- 1 banana
- Handful of spinach
- 1/2 cup Greek yogurt
- 1 tablespoon chia seeds
- 1 cup almond milk

Instructions:
1. Combine berries, banana, spinach, Greek yogurt, chia seeds, and almond milk in a blender.
2. Blend until smooth.
3. Pour into a glass and savor the energizing goodness.

2. Overnight Oats: A Time-Saving Marvel

Personal Insight: Mornings can be rushed, and the last thing I wanted was to spend precious moments preparing breakfast. Overnight oats became my morning savior – a grab-and-go option that packed a nutritional punch.

Ingredients for Chocolate Peanut Butter Overnight Oats:
- 1/2 cup rolled oats
- 1/2 cup milk of your choice
- 1 tablespoon cocoa powder
- 1 tablespoon peanut butter
- 1 tablespoon honey
- Sliced bananas for topping

Instructions:
1. In a jar, combine rolled oats, milk, cocoa powder, peanut butter, and honey.

2. Stir well, ensuring all ingredients are thoroughly mixed.

3. Refrigerate overnight.

4. In the morning, top with sliced bananas and relish the decadent simplicity.

3. Energizing Egg Muffins: Protein-Packed Bites

Personal Insight: Protein was a morning essential for me, but cooking a full breakfast seemed like a daunting task. Enter the energizing egg muffins – a portable, protein-packed delight that made mornings a breeze.

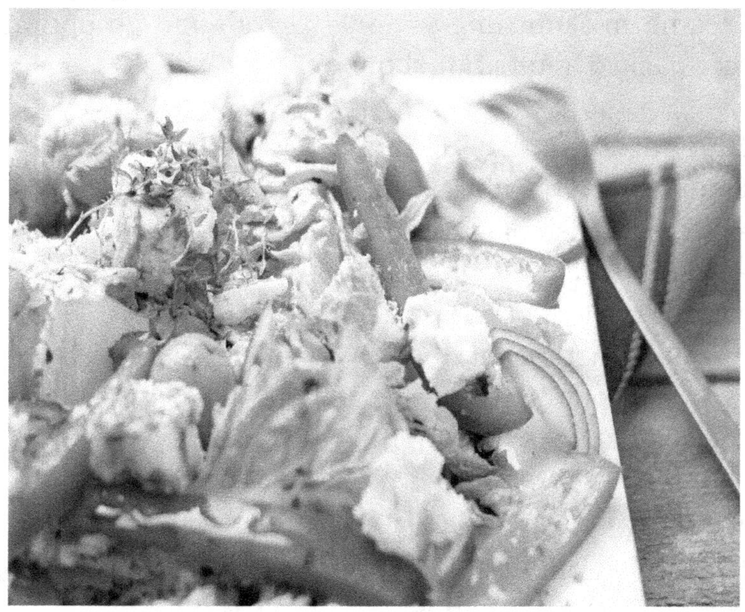

Ingredients for Veggie Egg Muffins:
- 6 eggs
- 1/2 cup bell peppers, diced
- 1/2 cup spinach, chopped
- 1/4 cup feta cheese, crumbled
- Salt and pepper to taste

Instructions:
1. Preheat the oven to 375°F (190°C).
2. In a bowl, whisk together eggs, diced bell peppers, chopped spinach, feta cheese, salt, and pepper.
3. Spoon mixture into muffin tray that has been buttered.
4. Bake for 15-20 minutes or until the egg muffins are set.

4. Nut Butter Banana Toast: Simple and Satisfying

Personal Insight: Some mornings, simplicity was key. Nut butter banana toast became my go-to – a delightful combination of creamy, crunchy, and naturally sweet.

Ingredients:
- 2 slices whole-grain bread
- Nut butter of your choice (almond, peanut, or cashew)

- 1 banana, sliced

Instructions:

1. Toast the whole-grain bread slices.
2. Spread a generous layer of nut butter on each slice.
3. Top with banana slices.
4. Enjoy the satisfying crunch and sweetness.

5. Greek Yogurt Parfait: Layers of Goodness

Personal Insight: This breakfast booster was not just a feast for the taste buds but also a visual delight. Layering Greek yogurt with fruits and granola elevated my mornings to a mini celebration.

Ingredients:
- 1 cup Greek yogurt
- 1/2 cup mixed berries
- 1/4 cup granola
- Drizzle of honey

Instructions:

1. In a glass or bowl, layer Greek yogurt, mixed berries, and granola.
2. Repeat the layers until the container is filled.
3. Drizzle honey over the top for a touch of sweetness.

In Conclusion: A Breakfast Symphony of Nourishment

As you navigate the delicate balance of mornings during pregnancy, consider these breakfast boosters as your allies. They are not just recipes; they are moments of self-care and nourishment, setting the stage for a day filled with energy and well-being.

Here's to breakfasts that go beyond sustenance – mornings infused with the symphony of vitality and joy.

CHAPTER 3 -
SECOND TRIMESTER NUTRIENT BOOST TIME

As you transition to the second trimester, your baby's growth accelerates, and so do your nutritional needs. Let's focus on practical tips for this stage:

1. Iron, Calcium, and Protein: These become the nutritional superheroes. Lean meats, dairy or fortified plant-based milk, and protein-rich foods like eggs and legumes should find a regular place on your plate.

2. Explore New Foods: Your taste buds may be changing, and that's perfectly normal. Embrace the opportunity to explore new foods and find what satisfies your evolving palate.

3. Moderate Exercise: Consider incorporating moderate exercise into your routine, with your healthcare provider's approval. It can boost your energy levels and contribute to a healthy pregnancy.

NUTRIENT- RICH MEALS FOR BABY'S GROWTH

Welcoming a new life into the world is a joyous occasion, and providing your baby with the best nutrition is a crucial part of ensuring healthy growth and development. Let's explore some straightforward and practical tips for preparing nutrient-rich meals that support your baby's growth in their early months.

1. Breastfeeding: Nature's Perfect Nutrition

Why Breastfeed:
Breast milk is a powerhouse of nutrients perfectly designed for your baby. It provides essential antibodies, proteins, fats, and carbohydrates crucial for their growth and immune system development.

Practical Tip 1: Establish a Comfortable Routine
Establishing a consistent breastfeeding routine can help both you and your baby. Find a comfortable and quiet place, and allow your baby to nurse whenever they show signs of hunger.

Practical Tip 2: Stay Hydrated and Well-Nourished

Remember to stay hydrated and nourished yourself. Your well-being directly impacts the quality of your breast milk. Aim for a balanced diet with a variety of fruits, vegetables, whole grains, and proteins.

2. Introduction to Solid Foods

When to Start Solids:
Around six months, your baby will show signs of readiness for solid foods, such as sitting up on their own and showing interest in what you're eating.

Practical Tip 3: Start with Single-Ingredient Foods

When introducing solids, begin with single-ingredient purees like mashed bananas, sweet potatoes, or peas. This aids in determining any possible sensitivities or allergies.

Practical Tip 4: Gradual Introduction of Allergenic Foods

As your baby gets older, consider introducing allergenic foods like peanuts, eggs, and dairy.Start with tiny doses and keep an eye out for any negative effects.

3. Creating Nutrient-Rich Puree

Avocado and Banana Puree:
- 1 ripe avocado
- 1 ripe banana

Instructions:
1. Mash the avocado and banana together until smooth.
2. Adjust the texture by adding breast milk or formula if needed.

Why It Works:
Avocados are rich in healthy fats, while bananas provide natural sweetness and potassium.

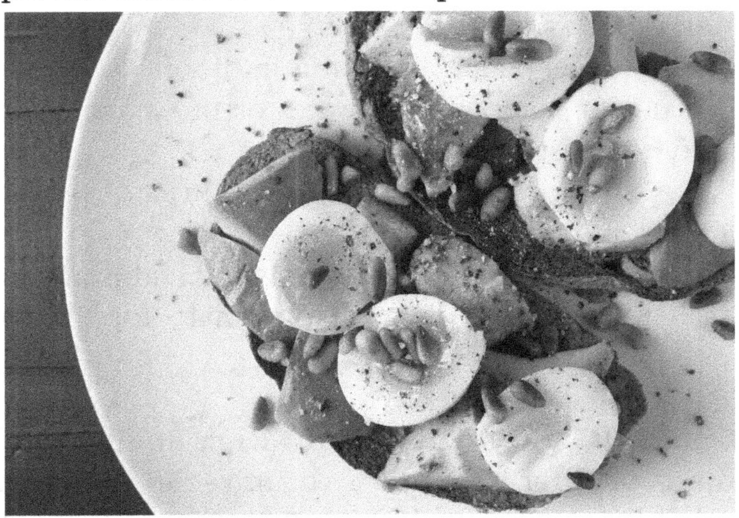

Practical Tip 5: Introduce a Variety of Textures

As your baby becomes more accustomed to solids, gradually introduce thicker textures. This helps develop their oral motor skills and prepares them for a variety of foods.

4. Iron-Rich Meals for Brain Development

Sweet Potato and Lentil Puree:
- 1 sweet potato, peeled and diced
- 1/2 cup red lentils, rinsed

Instructions:
1. Steam sweet potato and lentils until soft.
2. Blend together, adding water or breast milk for desired consistency.

Why It Works:
Sweet potatoes provide vitamin A, and lentils are an excellent source of iron, crucial for brain development.

Practical Tip 6: Include Iron-Rich Foods
Iron is vital for your baby's cognitive development. Include iron-rich foods like meats, legumes, and fortified cereals in their diet.

5. Finger Foods for Developing Motor Skills

Steamed Broccoli Florets:
- Fresh broccoli florets

Instructions:
1. Steam broccoli until tender but still firm.
2. Allow it to cool before serving.

Why It Works:
Broccoli is packed with vitamins and minerals. Offering finger foods encourages self-feeding and helps develop fine motor skills.

Practical Tip 7: Practice Safe Self-Feeding
Supervise your baby closely during self-feeding and avoid small, choking hazards. Cut foods into small, manageable pieces and encourage them to explore different textures.

6. Yogurt Parfait for Calcium and Probiotics

Ingredients:
- Full-fat plain yogurt
- Mashed berries
- Crushed graham crackers

Instructions:
1. Layer yogurt, mashed berries, and crushed graham crackers.
2. Serve in a small, baby-friendly bowl.

Why It Works:
Yogurt provides calcium for strong bones, and the probiotics support a healthy digestive system.

Practical Tip 8: Choose Full-Fat Dairy
In the early years, babies need the extra fat for brain development. Choose full-fat dairy products over low-fat or fat-free options.

7. Homemade Baby Oatmeal

Ingredients:
- 1/4 cup old-fashioned oats
- 1/2 cup water or breast milk
- Mashed banana (optional)
- Cinnamon (optional)

Instructions:
1. Cook oats with water or breast milk until soft.
2. Mix in mashed banana and a sprinkle of cinnamon if desired.

Why It Works:
Oats provide fiber and essential nutrients, and bananas add natural sweetness.

Practical Tip 9: Gradually Introduce Spices
Introduce mild spices like cinnamon or nutmeg to expand your baby's palate.
Start with little sums and see how they react.

In Conclusion

Nourishing your baby doesn't have to be complicated. Simple, homemade recipes using nutrient-rich ingredients lay a solid foundation for their growth and development. Whether you're breastfeeding or introducing solids, paying attention to your baby's cues and gradually incorporating a variety of foods can make the journey enjoyable and nutritious. Remember, every baby is different, so be flexible, and most importantly, savor the precious moments of watching your little one grow.

BALANCING CRAVINGS AND NUTRITIONAL NEEDS

The delicate dance of pregnancy cravings – a waltz between the desires of the palate and the needs of your growing baby. In this chapter, we'll explore the art of balance, offering practical tips to navigate the cravings with a touch of nutritional finesse.

Understanding the Craving Conundrum:

Cravings during pregnancy are as common as baby kicks and late-night bathroom visits. The key is not to resist them but to find a harmonious coexistence with your nutritional goals.

1. Embrace the Craving, Don't Fight It:

Cravings are like the friendly companions of pregnancy. Instead of viewing them as adversaries, embrace them. Acknowledge the craving, and let it be a part of your culinary journey. Cravings are often your body's way of signaling a need for specific nutrients.

Personal Insight: During my pregnancy, I craved chocolate like it held the secrets of the universe.

Rather than resisting, I opted for dark chocolate with nuts – a satisfying compromise that contributed both pleasure and nutritional value.

2. Find Nutrient-Rich Alternatives:

Craving sweets? Instead of reaching for processed candies, consider naturally sweet options. Fresh fruits, yogurt with honey, or a homemade fruit smoothie can satiate your sweet tooth while providing essential vitamins.

Craving something salty? Opt for nuts, seeds, or whole-grain crackers. These choices not only address the salt craving but also deliver healthy fats and fiber.

Personal Insight: When my salt cravings hit, I discovered the joy of roasted chickpeas. They satisfied the crunch and saltiness while offering a protein boost.

3. Opt for Balanced Combos:

Create balanced combinations that encompass both the craving and nutritional elements. If you're yearning for something indulgent, consider whole-grain toast with nut butter or a small serving of cheese with whole-grain crackers.

Personal Insight: When my craving whispered the desire for a savory indulgence, I crafted a delightful combination of whole-grain crackers with cheese. It became a mini-celebration of satisfaction and nourishment.

4. Mindful Indulgence:

Indulgence is not a dirty word; it's about enjoying your cravings in moderation. Instead of completely denying yourself, practice mindful indulgence. Savor each bite, be present in the moment, and relish the flavors.

Personal Insight: Craving a creamy treat led me to discover the joy of Greek yogurt with a drizzle of honey. It became a delightful ritual – a moment of sweetness without the guilt.

5. Stay Hydrated:

Sometimes, cravings are a result of dehydration rather than a genuine desire for a specific food. Before reaching for that craving, have a glass of water. Hydration can often curb the intensity of the craving.

Personal Insight: When a sudden craving for something sweet struck, I started with a glass of water. Surprisingly, the craving often diminished, revealing that my body was subtly asking for hydration.

In Conclusion: A Symphony of Balance:

Balancing cravings and nutritional needs during pregnancy is like conducting a symphony – each note contributing to the beautiful composition of your journey. Remember, cravings are not your adversaries; they are the gentle nudges guiding you towards your body's unique needs.

As you waltz through the cravings, find joy in the balance – the sweet with the nutritious, the salty with the wholesome. Let each craving be a part of the melody, creating a harmonious rhythm in your pregnancy journey.

Here's to the art of balancing cravings and nutritional needs – a delightful dance that celebrates both pleasure and nourishment.

Nourishing Lunches: Fueling Your Afternoons

The midday hours call for a lunch that not only satisfies hunger but also replenishes energy for the tasks ahead. In this chapter, I'll share nourishing lunches that became my go-to during pregnancy, offering a blend of flavors, nutrients, and the comfort needed to power through the afternoon. Join me in exploring these lunchtime delights that turn nourishment into a daily celebration.

1. Quinoa and Chickpea Buddha Bowl: A Wholesome Feast

Personal Insight: This Buddha bowl became my lunchtime ritual — a colorful symphony of textures and flavors. Quinoa provided a protein boost, while chickpeas contributed fiber and essential minerals. The vibrant medley of vegetables made each bite a celebration of nourishment.

Ingredients:
- 1 cup cooked quinoa
- 1/2 cup cooked chickpeas
- Mixed vegetables, including bell peppers, cucumbers, and cherry tomatoes.
- Avocado, sliced
- Hummus for dressing
- Fresh herbs for garnish

Instructions:
1. Arrange cooked quinoa at the base of the bowl.
2. Add cooked chickpeas, mixed vegetables, and sliced avocado.
3. Drizzle with hummus as a dressing.
4. Garnish with fresh herbs for a burst of flavor.

2. Lentil and Vegetable Soup: Hearty Comfort in a Bowl

Personal Insight: Some days called for warmth and simplicity. This lentil and vegetable soup became my bowl of comfort – a hearty hug in liquid form. The combination of lentils and vegetables provided a wholesome blend of protein and vitamins.

Ingredients:
- 1 cup lentils, rinsed
- Mixed vegetables (carrots, celery, onion, kale)
- Vegetable broth
- Garlic and herbs for flavor
- Salt and pepper to taste

Instructions:
1. 1. Saute the onions and garlic in a saucepan until aromatic.
2. Add mixed vegetables and lentils.
3. Add the veggie broth and heat through.
4. Season with herbs, salt, and pepper.
5. Simmer until lentils are tender.

3. **Grilled Chicken Salad**: Crisp and Satisfying

Personal Insight: This grilled chicken salad was a lunchtime favorite, offering a delightful mix of crunch and protein. The grilled chicken added a savory note, and the assortment of fresh vegetables made it a satisfying and nutrient-packed meal.

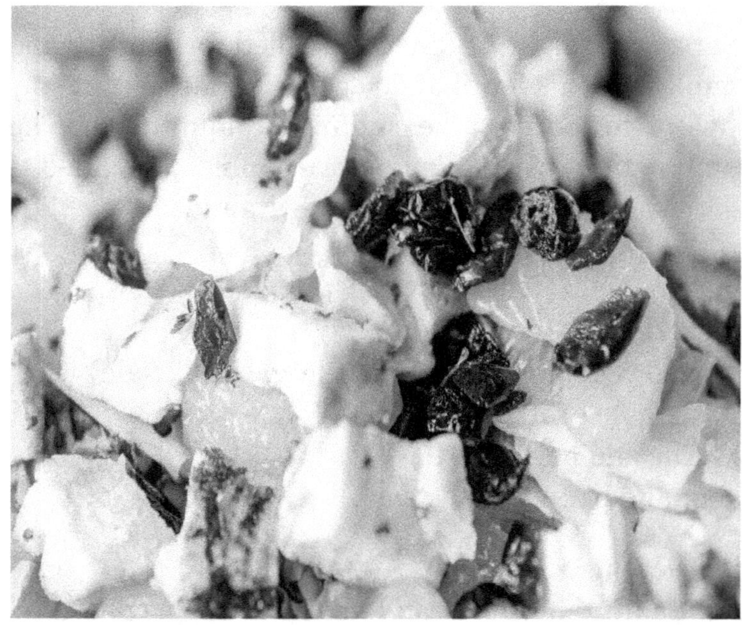

Ingredients:
- Grilled chicken breast, sliced
- Mixed salad greens
- Cherry tomatoes, halved
- Cucumber, sliced

- Feta cheese, crumbled
- Balsamic vinaigrette for dressing

Instructions:
1. Spoon a platter with mixed salad greens.
2. Top with grilled chicken slices, cherry tomatoes, cucumber, and crumbled feta cheese.
3. Drizzle with balsamic vinaigrette for a burst of flavor.

4. Sweet Potato and Black Bean Wrap: A Flavorful Wrap-and-Go

Personal Insight: When time was of the essence, this sweet potato and black bean wrap came to the rescue. The combination of sweet potatoes and black beans provided a satisfying fusion of sweetness and earthiness, all wrapped up for a convenient, nourishing lunch.

Ingredients:
- Whole-grain wrap or tortilla
- Roasted sweet potatoes, sliced
- Black beans, cooked
- Avocado, mashed
- Salsa for topping

Instructions:
1. First, place the whole-grain wrapper on a level area.

2. Spread mashed avocado along the center.
3. Add roasted sweet potatoes, black beans, and salsa.
4. Fold the sides of the wrap and enjoy.

5. Quinoa Salad with Lemon-Tahini Dressing: Zesty Elegance

Personal Insight: This quinoa salad became my go-to for a light yet satisfying lunch. The lemon-tahini dressing added a zesty elegance to the nutty quinoa, making it a refreshing and nutrient-rich choice.

Ingredients:
- 1 cup cooked quinoa
- Mixed greens
- Cherry tomatoes, halved
- Cucumber, diced
- Red onion, finely chopped
- Feta cheese, crumbled

For the Dressing:
- 2 tablespoons tahini
- Juice of 1 lemon
- Olive oil
- Salt and pepper to taste

Instructions:

1. In a bowl, combine cooked quinoa, mixed greens, cherry tomatoes, cucumber, red onion, and feta cheese.
2. In a small bowl, whisk together tahini, lemon juice, olive oil, salt, and pepper.
3. Gently toss the salad after drizzling it with dressing.

In Conclusion: A Lunchtime Symphony of Nourishment

As you embark on your afternoon journey, let these nourishing lunches be more than just a meal. Consider them a symphony of flavors and nutrients, harmonizing to fuel your body and uplift your spirit.

Here's to lunches that nourish, energize, and turn the ordinary into a daily celebration.

CHAPTER 4:
THIRD TRIMESTER : FUELING THE FINISH LINE

As you enter the final stretch, your baby and your body are gearing up for the finish line. Here are practical tips for the third trimester:

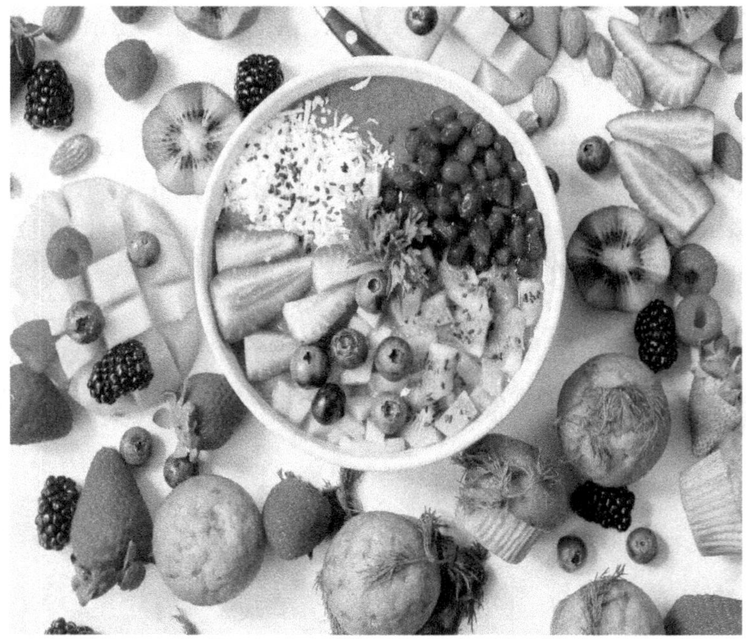

1. Protein and Omega-3 Fatty Acids: Maintain a focus on protein for your baby's growth and omega-3 fatty acids for brain development. Incorporate fish, nuts, and seeds into your meals.

2. Nutrient-Dense Snacking: Choose nutrient-dense snacks to keep your energy levels up. Think yogurt with fruit, a handful of nuts, or whole-grain crackers with cheese.

3. Hydrate, Hydrate, Hydrate: Staying hydrated is crucial, especially as your blood volume increases. Aim for at least eight glasses of water a day and consider hydrating foods like watermelon and cucumber.

Iron-Rich Recipes for Healthy Blood

I remember a time when I felt constantly fatigued and lacked the energy to tackle daily activities. Little did I know that my iron levels were taking a toll on my overall well-being. That realization led me on a journey to discover delicious and practical ways to incorporate iron-rich recipes into my diet, transforming my energy levels and promoting a healthier blood profile.

The Iron Connection: Why It Matters

Iron is like the unsung hero in our bodies. It plays a vital role in transporting oxygen through our blood, ensuring our muscles and organs get the oxygen they need to function optimally. When iron levels are low, fatigue, weakness, and even shortness of breath can become daily companions.

Unveiling the Iron-Rich Arsenal

1. Spinach and Chickpea Power Bowl

Spinach, a green powerhouse, meets the protein-packed chickpeas in this vibrant bowl.

Ingredients:
- 2 cups fresh spinach leaves

- 1 cup canned chickpeas, drained and rinsed
- 1 tablespoon olive oil
- 1 clove garlic, minced
- Salt and pepper to taste

Instructions:
1. Sauté minced garlic in olive oil until fragrant.
2. Add chickpeas to the pan and cook until golden brown.
3. Toss in fresh spinach and cook until wilted.
4. Season with salt and pepper.

Why It Works:
Spinach brings a hefty dose of non-heme iron, while chickpeas contribute both iron and protein. The garlic adds flavor and, surprisingly, a bit of an immune boost!

2. Beef and Broccoli Stir-Fry

Classic flavors meet a nutritional powerhouse in this quick and easy stir-fry.

Ingredients:
- 1 cup lean beef strips
- 2 cups broccoli florets
- 2 tablespoons soy sauce
- 1 tablespoon sesame oil
- 1 teaspoon grated ginger

Instructions:
1. Stir-fry beef strips until browned.
2. Add broccoli and cook until tender-crisp.
3. Mix soy sauce, sesame oil, and grated ginger.
4. Pour sauce over the beef and broccoli, toss until coated.

Why It Works:
Lean beef is a fantastic source of heme iron, which is easily absorbed by the body. The broccoli adds a boost of vitamin C, enhancing iron absorption.

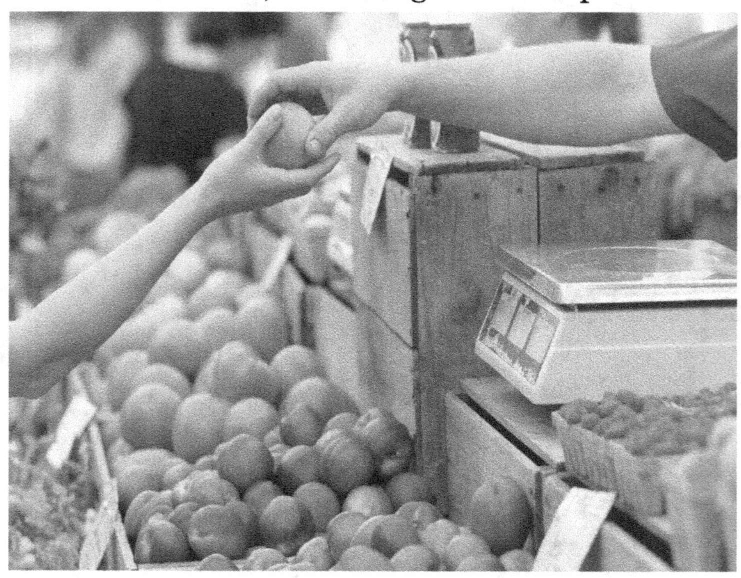

COOKING WITH PURPOSE : PRACTICAL TIPS

1. Pairing for Absorption

Iron comes in two forms: heme and non-heme. Heme iron, found in animal products, is more easily absorbed by the body. Non-heme iron, found in plant-based sources, can benefit from a little boost.

Practical Tip:
Pair non-heme iron sources with vitamin C-rich foods. For example, squeeze lemon juice over your spinach salad or toss some strawberries into your morning oatmeal.

2. Ditching the Culinary Myths

There's a common misconception that a vegetarian or vegan diet may lead to iron deficiency. While it's true that plant-based iron isn't as easily absorbed as heme iron, incorporating a variety of iron-rich plant foods and following the pairing tips can create a balanced and nourishing diet.

Practical Tip:
Blend black beans into a smooth hummus with a sprinkle of vitamin C-rich paprika for a tasty iron-packed dip.

PERSONAL EXPERIENCE : FROM FATIGUE TO VITALITY

As I began to integrate these iron-rich recipes into my meals, the transformation was astounding. The constant fatigue lifted, and my energy levels soared. It was more than just a change in diet; it was a change in lifestyle.

I realized that nourishing my body with the right foods was like giving it a secret weapon against exhaustion. The Spinach and Chickpea Power Bowl became a lunchtime favorite, providing a perfect balance of iron and protein to power me through the afternoon.

The Beef and Broccoli Stir-Fry, on the other hand, was my go-to for busy weeknight dinners. Quick, delicious, and loaded with heme iron from the beef, it made me feel like I was treating myself while still taking care of my nutritional needs.

Conclusion: Iron-Rich Living

As I share my personal journey, I encourage you to embark on your own exploration of iron-rich recipes. Whether you're a fan of spinach or beef, or perhaps both, the key is to find what works for you and fits seamlessly into your lifestyle.

Iron-rich living isn't about restriction; it's about abundance. Abundant energy, abundant vitality, and an abundant array of delicious foods that support your body in its journey to maintain healthy blood.

So, try the recipes, embrace the tips, and savor the experience of cooking with purpose. Your body will thank you, not only with increased energy but with an overall sense of well-being that comes from providing it with the nutrients it craves. Cheers to a life fueled by the power of iron!

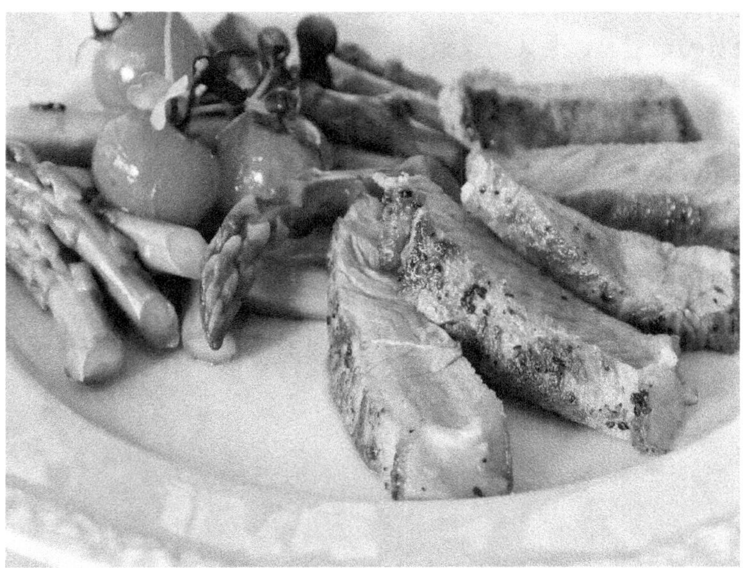

Calcium-Packed Dishes for Strong Bones

Picture this: a time when every step felt like a challenge, and I found myself constantly worrying about the health of my bones. That's when I discovered the transformative power of calcium-packed dishes. Not only did they bring flavor to my plate, but they also brought strength to my bones, allowing me to step into each day with confidence. Let's delve into the world of calcium-rich recipes that made a significant impact on my bone health.

The Calcium Connection: A Vital Ingredient for Strong Bones

Calcium is like the superhero of bone health. It's the mineral that forms the backbone of our skeletal system, literally. As we age, maintaining an adequate calcium intake becomes crucial to prevent bone loss and ensure our bones remain sturdy and resilient.

Unleashing the Calcium Heroes

1. Cheesy Spinach and Mushroom Stuffed Chicken Breast

This dish not only satisfies your taste buds but also provides a hefty dose of calcium.

Ingredients:
- 2 boneless, skinless chicken breasts
- 1 cup fresh spinach, chopped
- 1/2 cup mushrooms, finely diced
- 1/2 cup mozzarella cheese, shredded
- Salt, pepper, and your favorite herbs

Instructions:
1. Butterfly the chicken breasts.
2. Sauté spinach and mushrooms until cooked.
3. Mix cooked spinach, mushrooms, and cheese.
4. Stuff the chicken breasts with the mixture and secure with toothpicks.
5. Season with salt, pepper, and herbs.
6. Bake until the chicken is cooked through.

Why It Works:
Apart from the obvious calcium boost from the cheese, the spinach adds vitamin K, which is essential for bone health, and the mushrooms contribute vitamin D, aiding calcium absorption.

2. Creamy Broccoli and Cheddar Soup

Warm, comforting, and an excellent source of calcium.

Ingredients:
- 2 cups broccoli florets
- 1 cup sharp cheddar cheese, shredded
- 1 onion, diced
- 2 cloves garlic, minced
- 2 cups vegetable or chicken broth
- 1 cup milk (dairy or plant-based)

Instructions:
1. Sauté onions and garlic until soft.
2. Add broccoli and broth, simmer until broccoli is tender.
3. Blend the mixture until smooth.
4. Return to heat, add cheese and milk, stir until melted.
5. Season to taste.

Why It Works:
Broccoli brings calcium to the table, and the cheddar cheese not only adds creaminess but also a hefty dose of bone-strengthening calcium.

COOKING WITH PURPOSE : PRACTICAL TIPS

1. Beyond Dairy: Exploring Non-Dairy Calcium Sources

While dairy products are a classic source of calcium, it's essential to recognize that other foods can contribute significantly to your calcium intake.

Practical Tip:
Incorporate more plant-based sources of calcium, like tofu, almonds, and fortified plant milks, into your diet. These options not only diversify your meals but also cater to different dietary preferences.

2. The Calcium-Magnesium Duo

Calcium and magnesium work hand in hand to keep our bones in top-notch condition. While calcium builds bones, magnesium helps the body effectively utilize calcium.

Practical Tip:
Include magnesium-rich foods like nuts, seeds, and whole grains in your meals. This synergistic approach ensures that your body maximizes the benefits of the calcium you consume.

Personal Experience: From Fragility to Resilience

In the moments when I felt like my bones were fragile, I turned to these calcium-packed dishes as a form of self-care. The Cheesy Spinach and Mushroom Stuffed Chicken Breast became a symbol of nourishment, both for my taste buds and my bones. The calcium-rich cheese melded seamlessly with the savory mushrooms, creating a dish that was as comforting as it was nutritious.

The Creamy Broccoli and Cheddar Soup, with its warmth and richness, became a go-to for chilly evenings. Knowing that each spoonful not only satisfied my craving for something hearty but also fortified my bones gave me a sense of empowerment.

Conclusion: A Life Rooted in Strength

As I share my personal journey, I encourage you to embark on your own exploration of calcium-packed dishes. It's not just about adding ingredients to your meals; it's about building a foundation of strength that supports you through every step, every day.

Calcium-packed dishes aren't just about preventing bone issues; they're about embracing a lifestyle that values and cares for your bones. So, savor the Cheesy

Spinach and Mushroom Stuffed Chicken Breast, cozy up with a bowl of Creamy Broccoli and Cheddar Soup, and feel the strength and resilience that comes from nourishing your bones with purpose. Here's to a life rooted in strength, one delicious and calcium-rich meal at a time!

FOODS TO BOOST ENERGY AND STAMINA

We've all been there – those days when fatigue seems to be our constant companion, and every task feels like a marathon. The good news is that a simple shift in your diet can make a world of difference. Let's explore some straightforward and practical tips on foods that can boost your energy and stamina, helping you power through your day with vitality.

The Energy Equation: Fueling Your Body Right

Understanding the basics of how our bodies derive energy can help us make informed choices about the foods we eat. Energy comes from the food we consume, and the three main macronutrients – carbohydrates, proteins, and fats – play key roles in this process.

1. Carbohydrates: The Instant Energy Source

Carbohydrates are like fast fuel for your body. They break down into glucose, providing a quick source of energy. Opt for complex carbohydrates that release energy gradually, sustaining your stamina.

Practical Tip 1: Include Whole Grains**Replace processed grains with whole grains such as oats, brown rice, and quinoa. These grains contain more fiber, keeping you fuller for longer and providing sustained energy.

Practical Tip 2: Snack on Fruits
Fruits offer natural sugars and fiber. Snack on a banana or apple for a quick energy boost without the crash that comes with sugary snacks.

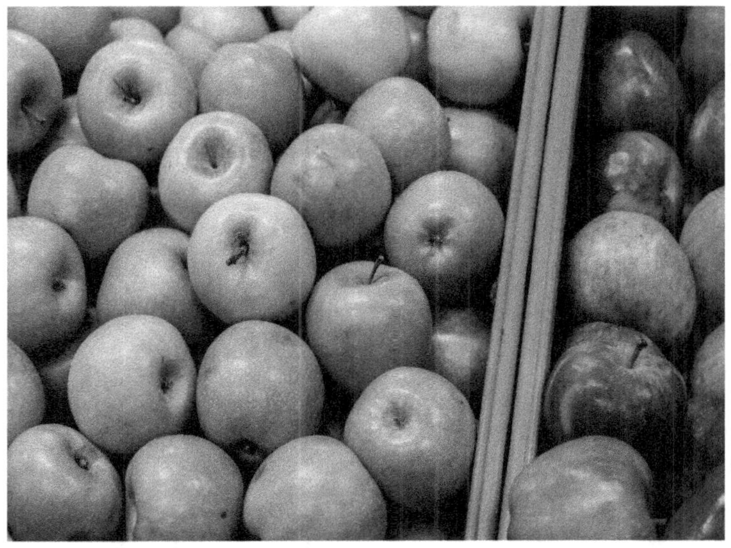

2. Proteins: The Building Blocks for Endurance

Proteins are crucial for repairing tissues and building muscle. Including protein in your meals helps sustain energy levels and prevents the feeling of fatigue.

Practical Tip 3: Prioritize Lean Proteins**
Pick lean protein sources such as fish, poultry, lentils, and beans. These options are lower in saturated fats and provide the essential amino acids your body needs.

Practical Tip 4: Combine Proteins with Carbs
Create balanced meals by pairing proteins with complex carbohydrates. For example, have grilled chicken with quinoa or beans with brown rice.There is a consistent discharge of energy from this combo.

3. Fats: The Sustained Energy Reservoir

While often misunderstood, fats are an essential part of a well-rounded diet. Healthy fats provide a concentrated source of energy and support various bodily functions.

Practical Tip 5: Choose Healthy Fats
Opt for sources of healthy fats like avocados, nuts, seeds, and olive oil. These fats provide a sustained release of energy and help you feel fuller for longer.

Practical Tip 6: Snack on Nut Mixes
Prepare a mix of nuts and seeds for a handy, energy-boosting snack. The combination of healthy fats and protein can keep you fueled throughout the day.

Personal Experience: From Sluggish to Energized

I vividly remember the days when a mid-afternoon slump would hit me like a ton of bricks. It felt like I was dragging my feet through every task, and productivity was a distant dream. It wasn't until I made some simple changes to my diet that I experienced a noticeable shift in my energy levels.

I started incorporating whole grains like quinoa and brown rice into my meals, bidding farewell to the quick energy crashes that came with refined grains. Snacking on fruits, especially bananas, became my go-to solution for a natural energy boost without the guilt of sugary snacks.

The inclusion of lean proteins, such as grilled chicken or chickpeas, brought a newfound endurance to my day. I no longer felt the need to reach for excessive caffeine to power through, as the combination of proteins and carbohydrates kept me steady and focused.

Practical Tips for Incorporating Energy-Boosting Foods

1. Hydration: The Foundation of Energy

Water is often underestimated when it comes to maintaining energy levels. Fatigue and lethargic sensations might result from dehydration.

Practical Tip 7: Drink Water Throughout the Day**
Make a habit of sipping water consistently throughout the day. Carry a reusable water bottle to ensure you stay hydrated, supporting overall energy levels.

2. Small, Frequent Meals: Steady Energy Release

Consider dividing your day into smaller, more frequent meals rather than three large ones. This approach helps maintain steady blood sugar levels, preventing energy dips.

Practical Tip 8: Plan Snacks Ahead
Prepare healthy snacks like yogurt with berries, carrot sticks with hummus, or a handful of nuts. Having these snacks readily available makes it easier to make nourishing choices.

3. Mindful Eating: Listening to Your Body

Observe the signals your body sends when it is hungry or full. Eating mindfully helps you make better food choices and prevents overeating, which can lead to feelings of sluggishness.

Practical Tip 9: Eat Slowly and Enjoy Your Food**
Take your time during meals. Eat slowly and thoroughly to fully appreciate the flavors. This not only aids digestion but also allows your body to signal when it's satisfied.

4. Incorporate Color: The Nutrient Powerhouses

Colorful fruits and vegetables are rich in vitamins and minerals, providing a natural energy boost. Try to arrange different hues on your plate.

Practical Tip 10: Build a Rainbow Plate**
Create visually appealing meals by incorporating a mix of colorful vegetables and fruits. Each color represents different nutrients, ensuring a diverse range of health benefits.

Conclusion: Energize Your Days, One Bite at a Time

Boosting your energy and stamina isn't about complicated diets or rigid meal plans. It's about making simple, sustainable changes to your daily eating habits. By incorporating a balance of carbohydrates, proteins, and healthy fats, staying hydrated, and practicing mindful eating, you can fuel your body for optimal performance.

As I reflect on my journey from sluggish to energized, I realize the profound impact that food choices can have on our daily lives. So, the next time you feel the afternoon slump creeping in, reach for a whole-grain snack, savor a piece of lean protein, or hydrate with a refreshing glass of water. Energize your days, one bite at a time, and embrace the vitality that comes with nourishing your body with purpose.

CHAPTER 5:
SNACKS AND TREATS FOR EVERY TRIMESTER

Pregnancy is a journey filled with cravings, changes, and the occasional hunger pangs. Navigating snacks and treats for each trimester can be a delightful experience. Here's a guide to satisfying your cravings while nourishing yourself during this special time.

First Trimester: Navigating Nausea

The first trimester can be a rollercoaster, especially when it comes to food. Nausea might be a constant companion, making it essential to choose snacks that are easy on the stomach.

Practical Tip 1: Ginger Delights
For a long time, ginger has been praised as a nausea cure. Try ginger tea, ginger snaps, or ginger candies for a soothing and flavorful relief.

Practical Tip 2: Crackers and Cheese
Keep some plain crackers and mild cheese on hand. The combination provides a good balance of carbohydrates and protein, and the mild flavors are less likely to trigger nausea.

Second Trimester: Energy Boosters

As your energy levels stabilize, the second trimester is an excellent time to focus on nutrient-dense snacks that keep you fueled and satisfied.

Practical Tip 3: Trail Mix
Combine a variety of nuts, seeds, and dried fruits to make a trail mix. It's a convenient and energy-boosting snack that can be easily customized to your taste.

Practical Tip 4: Greek Yogurt Parfait
Layer Greek yogurt with granola and fresh berries for a tasty and protein-packed treat. The calcium in yogurt is also beneficial for your growing baby's bones.

Third Trimester: Supporting Stamina

As you approach the final stretch, it's crucial to include snacks that support your stamina and provide the necessary nutrients for you and your baby.

Practical Tip 5: Nut Butter and Banana Sandwich
Toast whole-grain bread, spread with almond or peanut butter, and top with banana slices. This

snack provides a blend of complex carbohydrates, protein, and good fats.

Practical Tip 6: Dark Chocolate and Nuts
Indulge in some dark chocolate paired with a handful of nuts. Dark chocolate contains antioxidants, and nuts provide a mix of protein and healthy fats.

General Tips for All Trimesters

1. Hydration is Key
Stay hydrated by sipping water throughout the day. For a cool twist, add a dash of cucumber or lemon.

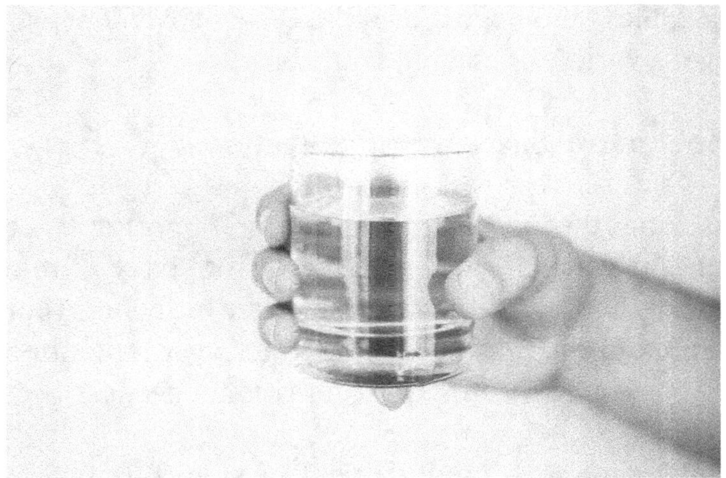

2. Listen to Your Cravings
While it's essential to nourish your body with healthy snacks, occasional indulgences are okay. If you're craving a treat, enjoy it in moderation.

3. Preparing Snacks in Advance
Plan ahead and have snacks readily available.
Pre-cut veggies, portion out trail mix, or have yogurt
cups in the fridge for quick and easy access.

4. Balanced Snacking
Opt for snacks that include a mix of carbohydrates,
proteins, and healthy fats. This balance helps keep
your energy levels stable and satisfies your hunger.

5. Smoothies for a Nutrient Boost
Blend up a nutrient-packed smoothie with fruits,
vegetables, and yogurt or milk. It's a convenient way
to get a variety of essential nutrients.

Conclusion: Snacking with Intention

Snacking during pregnancy is an opportunity to
nourish yourself and your growing baby. From
battling nausea in the first trimester to fueling your
stamina in the third, choosing snacks with intention
ensures you're meeting your nutritional needs.

So, whether it's a handful of nuts, a yogurt parfait, or
a treat to satisfy your sweet tooth, snack wisely and
enjoy every bite. Your body is working hard to
nurture new life, and these snacks are your delicious
companions on this incredible journey.

QUICK AND HEALTHY SNACK IDEAS

Life is fast-paced, and finding time for healthy snacks can be a challenge. But fear not! Nourishing your body with quick and healthy snacks doesn't have to be complicated. Let's explore some straightforward and delicious ideas to keep you energized throughout the day.

1. Greek Yogurt with Berries:
A classic that never gets old. Greek yogurt is rich in protein, and when paired with fresh berries, you get a delightful mix of vitamins, antioxidants, and a natural sweetness. It's a quick, no-fuss snack that satisfies your taste buds and keeps you full.

Practical Tip 1: Pre-portion Yogurt
To make this snack even more convenient, pre-portion yogurt into small containers and keep them in the fridge. Grab one when you need a quick pick-me-up.

2. Apple Slices with Nut Butter:
Slice up an apple and spread on some nut butter—whether it's almond, peanut, or cashew. The combination of crisp apples and creamy nut butter provides a perfect blend of fiber, healthy fats, and a touch of sweetness.

Practical Tip 2: Go for Nutrient-Rich Nut Butters
Select natural nut butters that don't have any added sugar or oil. These versions pack more nutrients and contribute to the overall health benefits of the snack.

 3. Vegetable Sticks with Hummus:
Chop up colorful veggies like carrots, cucumbers, and bell peppers, and dip them into hummus. This snack is not only crunchy and satisfying but also a great way to sneak in extra veggies.

Practical Tip 3: Prep Veggies in Advance
Take some time to chop and store veggies in the refrigerator at the beginning of the week. This makes it easy to grab a handful when hunger strikes.

 4. Trail Mix with a Twist:Put some nuts, seeds, and dried fruits in your trail mix. Add a sprinkle of dark chocolate or coconut flakes for extra flavor. Trail mix is portable and provides a balanced mix of protein, healthy fats, and carbohydrates.

Practical Tip 4: Portion Control
While trail mix is nutrient-dense, it's also calorie-dense. Portion out small servings to avoid mindless munching.

5. Whole Grain Crackers with Cheese:
Grab some healthy grain crackers and your preferred cheese to go with them. This snack offers a satisfying crunch along with a combination of fiber and protein.

Practical Tip 5: Experiment with Cheese Varieties
Try different types of cheese to keep things interesting. From creamy brie to sharp cheddar, there's a cheese for every palate.

6. Smoothie on the Go:
Blend up a quick smoothie with your favorite fruits, a handful of greens, and some yogurt or milk. It's a convenient way to get a variety of nutrients in one delicious drink.

Practical Tip 6: Freeze Fruits
Keep your favorite fruits in the freezer for an instant chill without the need for ice. Frozen fruits also add a refreshing texture to your smoothies.

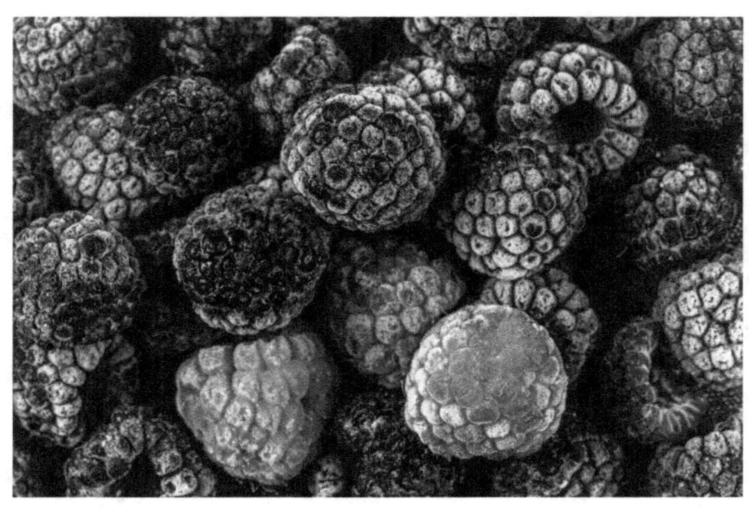

Conclusion: Snack Smart, Snack Simple

In the hustle and bustle of daily life, snacking often becomes an afterthought. However, with a little planning and creativity, you can make snacking a nourishing and enjoyable part of your routine. These quick and healthy snack ideas are not just about filling your stomach but about giving your body the nutrients it deserves.

So, whether you're at your desk, on the go, or simply relaxing at home, remember that a satisfying and healthy snack is just a few minutes away. Snack smart, snack simple, and let your energy soar!

INDULGENT YET NUTRITIOUS TREATS

Indulging in treats doesn't have to mean sacrificing your commitment to a healthy lifestyle. In fact, there are plenty of delicious and nutritious options that allow you to satisfy your sweet tooth without compromising on your well-being. Let's explore some practical tips for creating indulgent yet nutritious treats.

1. Choose Smart Ingredients:

When whipping up your favorite treats, opt for wholesome ingredients that pack a nutritional punch. Whole grains, nuts, seeds, and natural sweeteners like honey or maple syrup can add both flavor and nutritional value to your treats. These ingredients bring in essential nutrients, fiber, and healthy fats that contribute to your overall well-being.

2. Mindful Portion Control:

Enjoying treats in moderation is key to maintaining a balanced diet. Instead of devouring a whole batch of cookies, savor a couple and appreciate the flavors. Portion control allows you to indulge without going overboard on calories or sugar, helping you strike a healthy balance.

3. Incorporate Fruits:

Fruits are nature's candy, offering sweetness along with an array of vitamins and antioxidants. Incorporate fruits into your treats to enhance both flavor and nutritional content. Whether it's adding berries to yogurt, apple slices to muffins, or banana to pancakes, fruits elevate the taste while providing essential nutrients.

4. Swap Out Processed Sugars:

Opt for natural sweeteners over refined sugars. This simple swap can make a significant difference in the nutritional profile of your treats. Stevia, agave nectar, or date sugar are excellent alternatives that add sweetness without the drawbacks of processed sugars.

5. Experiment with Nut Butters:

Nut butters, such as almond or peanut butter, are not only delicious but also nutritious. They bring a rich and creamy texture to treats while providing healthy fats and protein. Try incorporating nut butters into your smoothies, cookies, or energy bites for a satisfying treat.

6. Bake, Don't Fry:

If you're into making treats like doughnuts or pastries, consider baking instead of frying. Baking reduces the amount of added fats, making your treats lighter and healthier. Plus, it's a simpler and less messy process, making it a win-win for both your taste buds and your health.

7. Dark Chocolate Delights:
When it comes to chocolatey indulgence, choose dark chocolate with higher cocoa content. Dark chocolate is rich in antioxidants and has less sugar compared to milk chocolate. Enjoy a small piece to satisfy your sweet cravings without overloading on sugar.

8. Mindful Dessert Choices:
Be mindful of the desserts you choose when dining out. Opt for options that incorporate fruits, nuts, or whole grains. Many restaurants now offer healthier dessert alternatives that allow you to treat yourself without compromising your commitment to a nutritious diet.

Remember, the key to indulgent yet nutritious treats lies in making thoughtful ingredient choices and practicing moderation. By incorporating these practical tips, you can enjoy delicious treats guilt-free while supporting your overall health and well-being.

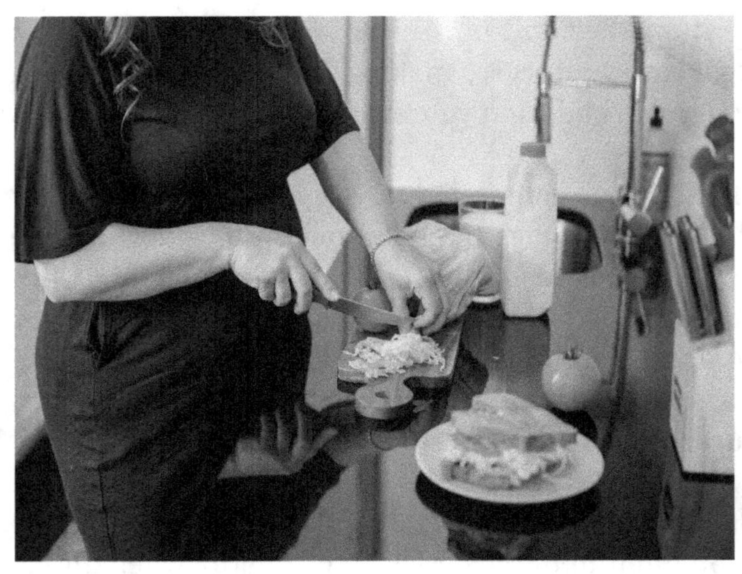

CRAVING -BUSTING OPTIONS

We've all been there — the sudden craving for something sweet, salty, or downright indulgent. Instead of succumbing to unhealthy options, let's explore some practical and nutritious alternatives to bust those cravings without compromising your well-being.

1. Sweet Tooth Solutions:
When the sugar cravings hit, try opting for naturally sweet alternatives. Fresh fruits like berries, mangoes, or a juicy apple can satisfy your sweet tooth without the added sugars. For a creamy

indulgence, mix Greek yogurt with honey and top it with a sprinkle of nuts or granola. This not only satisfies your craving but also provides a dose of protein and healthy fats.

2. Salty Snack Swaps:
Craving something salty? Instead of reaching for those greasy potato chips, consider air-popped popcorn seasoned with a dash of your favorite herbs or nutritional yeast. If you're a fan of crunch, roasted chickpeas or a handful of mixed nuts can be a satisfying alternative. These options deliver the savory taste you crave along with beneficial nutrients like fiber and good fats.

3. Guilt-Free Chocolate Fixes:
Chocolate cravings are common, and fortunately, there are healthier options. Dark chocolate with a high cocoa content not only satisfies your chocolate cravings but also provides antioxidants. If you're feeling creative, dip strawberries or banana slices in melted dark chocolate for a delicious and nutritious treat. Just be mindful of portion sizes to keep the calorie intake in check.

4. Comforting Warm Beverages:
Sometimes, a craving is more about the experience than the actual taste. Instead of reaching for a calorie-laden hot chocolate, opt for herbal teas.

Peppermint, chamomile, or cinnamon-infused teas can be comforting and naturally sweet without the added sugars. Add a splash of almond milk for a creamy touch without the excess calories.

5. DIY Nut Butter Delights:
Nut butters are a rich and satisfying option for those craving something indulgent. Make your own nut butter at home using almonds, peanuts, or cashews. Spread it on whole-grain toast or apple slices for a nutritious snack that curbs your craving and provides a good dose of healthy fats, protein, and fiber.

6. Hydrate to Alleviate:
Sometimes, cravings can be a sign of dehydration. Try sipping a glass of water before reaching for a food . Infuse it with slices of lemon, cucumber, or mint for a refreshing twist. Staying hydrated not only helps curb unnecessary cravings but also supports overall health.

In conclusion, managing cravings doesn't have to mean sacrificing your health goals. By making thoughtful and nutritious choices, you can indulge in satisfying treats without guilt. Experiment with these alternatives to discover what works best for you, and remember that moderation is key to maintaining a balanced and healthy lifestyle.

CHAPTER 6:

POSTPARTUM RECOVERY

Congratulations! You've brought a beautiful bundle of joy into the world, and now it's time to embark on the transformative journey of postpartum recovery. As I share this chapter, I'll weave in my personal experience, hoping to provide insights that resonate with you and guide you through this incredible yet challenging period.

1. Physical Healing:
Let's start with the body – a miraculous vessel that has just undergone the incredible feat of childbirth. My personal journey involved a mix of exhaustion and wonder as my body recovered. It's crucial to remember that healing takes time. From sore muscles to perineal discomfort, every twinge is a testament to the incredible work your body has done.

Practical Tip: Prioritize rest. I learned that rest isn't a luxury; it's a necessity. Take short naps when you can, and don't hesitate to accept help from loved ones.

2. Emotional Rollercoaster:

Postpartum emotions are like a rollercoaster – thrilling, unpredictable, and occasionally terrifying. My personal experience was filled with moments of overwhelming love and joy, but there were also tears and moments of self-doubt. It's okay to feel a mix of emotions; your body and mind are adjusting to a new normal.

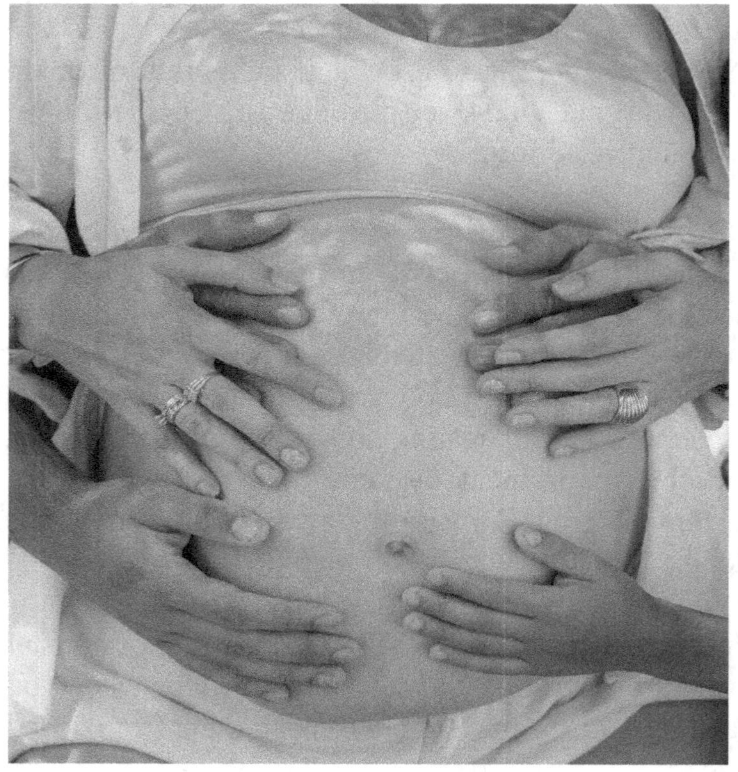

Practical Tip: Communicate. Share your feelings with your partner, friends, or a healthcare professional. You're not alone in this journey, and talking about your emotions can be incredibly cathartic.

3. Establishing a Support System:

During my postpartum recovery, I realized the importance of a strong support system. Whether it was my partner bringing me snacks during late-night feedings or a friend lending a listening ear, the support I received was invaluable. Lean on your loved ones – they want to help.

Practical Tip: Don't be afraid to ask for help. Whether it's assistance with household chores or someone to hold the baby while you take a shower, accept the support that's offered.

4. Navigating Sleep Deprivation:

The elusive concept of sleep after welcoming a newborn. My personal experience involved a dance of sleepless nights and daytime catnaps. While it's impossible to avoid sleep disruption entirely, finding moments to rest when the baby sleeps can make a significant difference.

Practical Tip: Sleep when the baby sleeps. It's a common piece of advice, and for a reason – it works. The laundry can wait; your well-being cannot.

5. Embracing the New Normal:
As I embraced my postpartum journey, I realized that my definition of normal was evolving. The days of spontaneous outings were replaced with a routine centered around the baby's needs. It's an adjustment, but it's also an opportunity to create a new, beautiful normal.

Practical Tip: Be patient with yourself. Embrace the changes, and understand that your 'normal' will continue to evolve as you and your baby grow together.

6. Celebrate Small Victories:
Postpartum recovery is a series of small victories. From the first time you manage a shower without interruption to conquering the challenge of a solo outing with the baby – celebrate these wins. My personal victories became cherished milestones in this incredible journey.

Practical Tip: Keep a journal. Documenting these small victories allows you to reflect on your progress and appreciate the resilience you discover within yourself.

In conclusion, postpartum recovery is a unique and transformative chapter in your life story. Embrace the physical changes, navigate the emotional landscape, and remember that you're not alone. Share your experiences, celebrate the victories, and, most importantly, savor the precious moments with your little one. You're stronger than you realize, and each day brings you closer to a stronger, wiser version of yourself.

Nourishing Your Body After Birth

Welcome to the postpartum journey, a time of joy, new beginnings, and undoubtedly, an array of unique challenges. As we explore the crucial aspect of nourishing your body after birth, I'll intertwine my personal experience, hoping to shed light on the importance of self-care during this transformative period.

1. Rebuilding from Within:
In the weeks following childbirth, my body felt like a warrior returning from battle – tired, resilient, and in need of restoration. Nourishing yourself now is not just about replenishing what was lost but about rebuilding your strength from within. Focus on nutrient-dense foods that support healing and energy.

Practical Tip: Embrace leafy greens, lean proteins, and whole grains. These foods provide essential vitamins and minerals, aiding in the recovery process.

2. Hydration is Key:
Amidst diaper changes and late-night feedings, it's easy to forget the simple act of sipping water. During my postpartum journey, I quickly realized the

importance of staying hydrated, especially if you're breastfeeding. Water is the unsung hero, promoting healing and assisting in milk production.

Practical Tip: Keep a water bottle handy, and set a goal to drink at least eight glasses of water a day. For an original perspective on refreshment, try herbal teas or infused water.

3. Snack Smartly:

With the unpredictable schedule of a newborn, regular meals might seem like a luxury. That's where smart snacking comes into play. My personal go-to snacks included nuts, yogurt, and fruit. These options are not only convenient but also packed with the nutrients your body craves.

*Practical Tip: Prepare snack packs in advance. Having a mix of healthy snacks readily available ensures you can refuel whenever hunger strikes.

4. Incorporate Omega-3 Fatty Acids:

As I navigated the postpartum period, I discovered the benefits of omega-3 fatty acids in supporting both physical and mental well-being. Fatty fish like salmon, flaxseeds, and walnuts became staples in my diet, promoting brain health and easing the post-baby blues.

Practical Tip: Include fatty fish in your meals at least twice a week or consider a fish oil supplement after consulting with your healthcare provider.

5. Listen to Your Body:
Postpartum nutrition is not a one-size-fits-all approach. Each body has different needs, and listening to your own cues is paramount. If you're craving a particular food, indulge in moderation. Your body may be signaling a need for specific nutrients.

Practical Tip: Keep a food journal to track how your body reacts to different foods. This can help you identify patterns and make informed choices that suit your individual needs.

6. Plan and Prepare:
In the whirlwind of new motherhood, finding time to cook elaborate meals can be challenging. I discovered the power of planning and preparing meals in advance. Whether it's a batch of hearty soup or pre-cut veggies for snacking, having nutritious options ready makes a world of difference.

Practical Tip: Set aside a dedicated time each week for meal prep. It doesn't have to be elaborate – simple, nourishing meals can be just as effective.

In conclusion, nourishing your body after birth is an essential component of your postpartum journey. As you embark on this chapter, remember that self-care is not a luxury but a necessity. Embrace the healing power of wholesome foods, stay hydrated, and allow yourself the grace to adapt to the changes. By prioritizing your well-being, you're not only caring for yourself but also laying the foundation for a healthy and vibrant future with your little one.

EASY AND QUICK RECIPES FOR NEW MOMS

Congratulations, new mom! Amidst the joy and chaos of motherhood, finding time to whip up nutritious meals can be a real challenge. Fear not, for this chapter is here to share some easy and quick recipes tailored to keep you well-fed and energized during this incredible journey.

1. Overnight Oats Powerhouse:
Start your day right with a simple yet nutritious breakfast – overnight oats. In a jar, combine rolled oats with your choice of milk, yogurt, and a dash of honey. Add your favorite toppings like sliced fruits, nuts, or seeds. Place the sealed jar in the refrigerator for the entire night. In the morning, voila! A delicious and nutrient-packed breakfast ready to enjoy.

Practical Tip: Prep multiple jars in advance for a hassle-free breakfast throughout the week.

2. Veggie-loaded Omelet:
When time is of the essence, a veggie-loaded omelet is your best friend. Whisk a couple of eggs, pour them into a hot, greased pan, and add diced vegetables like bell peppers, tomatoes, and spinach.

Fold it over, and within minutes, you have a protein-packed, veggie-loaded delight.

Practical Tip: Keep pre-chopped veggies in the fridge for even quicker preparation.

3. Avocado Toast with a Twist:
Elevate the classic avocado toast by adding extra layers of flavor. Mash ripe avocado on whole-grain toast and top it with cherry tomatoes, a sprinkle of feta cheese, and a drizzle of balsamic glaze. This tasty combination not only satisfies your taste buds but also provides essential nutrients.

Practical Tip: Experiment with various toppings like poached eggs or smoked salmon for added protein.

4. One-Pan Chicken and Veggies:
Dinner can be both quick and wholesome with a one-pan chicken and veggies dish. Toss chicken breast, chopped vegetables (think carrots, broccoli, and bell peppers), olive oil, and your favorite spices onto a baking sheet. Roast in the oven, and within 30 minutes, you have a balanced and delicious meal.

Practical Tip: Make extra to have leftovers for the next day.

5. Nut Butter Banana Wrap:
For a satisfying snack or a quick lunch, try a nut butter banana wrap. Spread your favorite nut butter

on a whole-grain tortilla, add sliced bananas, and perhaps a sprinkle of cinnamon. Roll it up, and you've got a tasty, energy-boosting treat.

Practical Tip: Customize with additions like chia seeds or a drizzle of honey for extra goodness.

6. Quick Quinoa Salad:
When you need a nutrient-packed meal in a flash, whip up a quick quinoa salad. Cook quinoa according to package instructions and toss it with cherry tomatoes, cucumber, feta cheese, and a simple olive oil and lemon dressing. This refreshing salad is not only quick to make but also perfect for satisfying hunger and providing essential nutrients.

Practical Tip: Prepare a larger batch and store it in the fridge for ready-to-go meals.

In conclusion, these easy and quick recipes for new moms are designed to simplify your mealtime without compromising on nutrition. Remember, it's okay to take shortcuts and make use of pre-cut veggies, frozen fruits, and other time-saving ingredients. The key is to nourish yourself efficiently so you can focus on the joys of motherhood without stressing about your plate. Happy cooking!

BUILDING NUTRIENT -RICH MEALS FOR BREASTFEEDING

As a new mom navigating the beautiful world of breastfeeding, ensuring you're getting the right nutrients is not just important for you but also for your little one. Let's explore some practical tips for building nutrient-rich meals that will keep both you and your baby well-nourished without the fuss.

1. Embrace the Power of Protein:
Protein is your ally in the breastfeeding journey, aiding in milk production and supporting your energy levels. Incorporate lean protein sources like chicken, turkey, fish, beans, lentils, and tofu into your meals. They're versatile and can be the star of a variety of dishes.

Practical Tip: Batch-cook protein sources ahead of time for quick and easy meal assembly.

2. Don't Skimp on Healthy Fats:
Healthy fats are crucial for brain development, and they also help keep you full and satisfied. Nuts, seeds, avocado, and olive oil are all great sources of good fats. Add a handful of nuts to your yogurt or drizzle olive oil over your veggies for a tasty boost.

Practical Tip: Keep a jar of mixed nuts or a small container of sliced avocado ready for snacking.

3. Load Up on Colorful Vegetables:
Vegetables are a treasure trove of vitamins and minerals. Try to load up half of your plate with different vibrant vegetables. Broccoli, carrots, bell peppers, and leafy greens not only provide essential nutrients but also add vibrant flavors and textures to your meals.

Practical Tip: Buy pre-cut veggies or chop them in batches for quick access.

4. Whole Grains for Sustained Energy:
Include entire grains in your meals, such as quinoa, brown rice, oats, and whole wheat bread. They provide complex carbohydrates that release energy slowly, helping you stay energized throughout the day.

Practical Tip: Cook extra whole grains and store them in the fridge for speedy meal assembly.

5. Include Calcium-Rich Foods:
Calcium is crucial for both you and your baby's bone health.Good sources of calcium include dairy

products, fortified plant-based milk, and leafy greens like collard greens and kale.

Practical Tip: Create a delicious smoothie by blending calcium-rich yogurt with fruits and a handful of spinach.

6. Stay Hydrated with Water and Hydrating Foods:

Breastfeeding can make you feel thirstier than usual. Make sure you consume enough water throughout the day to maintain proper hydration. Additionally, incorporate hydrating foods like watermelon, cucumber, and oranges into your meals.

Practical Tip: Carry a water bottle with you wherever you go to make hydration easy and accessible.

7. Plan Balanced Snacks:

Snacking is a breastfeeding mom's best friend. Plan snacks that balance protein, healthy fats, and carbohydrates. Greek yogurt with berries, a small handful of nuts, or a whole-grain cracker with cheese are excellent options.

Practical Tip: Prep snack boxes with a mix of nuts, dried fruits, and cheese for quick grabs.

In conclusion, building nutrient-rich meals for breastfeeding doesn't have to be complicated. Keep it simple, diverse, and enjoyable. Your body and your baby will thank you for the balanced and nourishing choices you make. Remember, there's no one-size-fits-all approach – listen to your body's cues, and don't hesitate to seek guidance from healthcare professionals for personalized advice. Happy and healthy breastfeeding!

CHAPTER 7:
SPECIAL DIETS AND CONSIDERATIONS

In the vast landscape of nutrition, there are instances where special diets become not just a choice but a necessity. Whether due to health conditions, personal preferences, or cultural considerations, navigating these dietary paths can seem challenging. Fear not, for this chapter aims to demystify special diets and provide practical tips for a smooth journey.

1. Gluten-Free Living:

For individuals with celiac disease or gluten sensitivity, embracing a gluten-free lifestyle is crucial. Fortunately, the food market now offers a variety of gluten-free alternatives. Swap regular flour with options like almond flour or coconut flour for baking. Experiment with gluten-free grains like quinoa, rice, and buckwheat for a wholesome diet.

Practical Tip: Check food labels for hidden sources of gluten, and consider consulting a dietitian for personalized guidance.

2. Plant-Based Bliss:

Whether motivated by ethical reasons or a desire for a healthful lifestyle, plant-based diets are gaining popularity. Opt for a variety of fruits, vegetables, legumes, nuts, and seeds to ensure a well-rounded intake of nutrients. Incorporate plant-based protein sources like tofu, lentils, and chickpeas into your meals for sustained energy.

Practical Tip: Plan meals ahead and explore plant-based recipes to keep your diet diverse and exciting.

3. Navigating Nut Allergies:

Nut allergies can be challenging, but with careful planning, a balanced diet is still achievable. Substitute nut butters with alternatives like sunflower seed butter or tahini. Explore nutrient-rich seeds like chia seeds, flaxseeds, and hemp seeds as valuable additions to your meals.

Practical Tip: Read food labels diligently, and inform restaurants about your nut allergy when dining out.

4. Managing Lactose Intolerance:

Lactose intolerance can affect your ability to digest dairy products. Fortunately, there are numerous lactose-free alternatives available, including almond milk, soy milk, and lactose-free yogurt. Incorporate calcium-rich foods like leafy greens, fortified plant-based milk, and tofu into your diet for bone health.

Practical Tip: Experiment with lactose-free dairy substitutes to find what suits your taste preferences.

5. Cultural Considerations:
Cultural and religious practices often play a significant role in dietary choices. Whether observing specific fasting periods, abstaining from certain foods, or following traditional culinary customs, it's essential to respect and adapt your diet accordingly. Explore alternative ingredients that align with your cultural dietary guidelines.

Practical Tip: Connect with communities that share similar dietary practices for inspiration and support.

6. Diabetic-Friendly Eating:
For those managing diabetes, maintaining stable blood sugar levels is paramount. Focus on whole, unprocessed foods, and opt for complex carbohydrates like whole grains and legumes. Prioritize lean proteins, healthy fats, and control portion sizes to help manage blood glucose levels effectively.

Practical Tip: Regularly monitor your blood sugar levels and work closely with healthcare professionals to tailor your diet to your specific needs.

7. Mindful Eating for Weight Management:
Sometimes, dietary considerations revolve around weight management goals. The key is to adopt a balanced, sustainable approach. Incorporate a variety of nutrient-dense foods, practice mindful eating, and stay physically active. Prioritize long-term habits over temporary solutions.

Practical Tip: Keep a food journal to track your eating patterns and identify areas for improvement.

8. FODMAP-Friendly Choices:
For those with irritable bowel syndrome (IBS), a low FODMAP diet may provide relief from digestive symptoms. This involves avoiding certain fermentable carbohydrates found in various foods. While navigating this diet, consider working with a dietitian to ensure you still achieve a well-balanced intake of nutrients.

Practical Tip: Gradually reintroduce FODMAPs to identify your personal tolerance levels.

9. Pregnancy and Breastfeeding Nutrition:
Special dietary considerations extend to pregnancy and breastfeeding. Nutrient needs change during these periods, requiring a focus on additional vitamins and minerals. Make sure you're getting enough calcium, iron, folic acid, and omega-3 fatty acids. Consulting with healthcare professionals can help tailor your diet to support a healthy pregnancy and breastfeeding journey.

Practical Tip: Take prenatal vitamins and maintain regular check-ins with healthcare providers to monitor your nutritional needs.

In conclusion, embarking on a special diet doesn't mean sacrificing flavor or nutrition. With thoughtful planning, a diverse range of foods can still be enjoyed, meeting specific dietary requirements. Whether it's gluten-free, plant-based, or tailored for health conditions, the key is to stay informed, experiment with new recipes, and seek guidance from healthcare professionals or dietitians when needed. Remember, your diet is a personal journey – make choices that align with your unique needs, preferences, and goals.

VEGETARIAN AND VEGAN PREGNANCY DIETS

Pregnancy is a time of immense joy and anticipation, and maintaining a balanced diet is crucial for both the health of the mother and the growing baby. For those following vegetarian or vegan lifestyles, it's entirely possible to meet all nutritional needs during this special time with thoughtful planning.

Nutritional Foundations:

A well-rounded vegetarian or vegan pregnancy diet centers on obtaining essential nutrients from plant-based sources. Key elements include:

1. Protein:
Protein is vital for fetal development. Ensure a variety of plant-based protein sources such as beans, lentils, tofu, tempeh, and quinoa. Additionally great additions to your diet are nuts and seeds.

2. Calcium:
Opt for fortified plant-based milk, tofu, leafy greens like kale and collard greens, and calcium-set tofu. These options can contribute to meeting your calcium requirements.

3. Iron:

Iron is crucial for preventing anemia. Incorporate iron-rich plant foods like lentils, beans, spinach, and fortified cereals.Iron absorption is improved when these are eaten with foods high in vitamin C.

4. Vitamin B12:

Vitamin B12 is primarily found in animal products, so it's essential for vegans to take supplements or consume fortified foods like plant-based milk, breakfast cereals, or nutritional yeast.

5. Omega-3 Fatty Acids:

Opt for plant-based sources of omega-3 fatty acids such as flaxseeds, chia seeds, walnuts, and algae-based supplements.

6. Folate:

Folate, crucial for preventing neural tube defects, is abundant in leafy greens, beans, lentils, and fortified cereals.

Practical Tips for a Balanced Vegetarian or Vegan Pregnancy Diet:

1. Diverse Protein Sources:

Include a variety of plant proteins to ensure you're getting a spectrum of amino acids. Beans, lentils, tofu, and tempeh offer a wide range of options to keep your diet interesting.

2. Calcium-Rich Choices:

Make conscious choices to incorporate calcium-rich foods. Fortified plant-based milk, fortified orange juice, and leafy greens can contribute significantly.

3. Iron Absorption Boosters:
Eat foods strong in vitamin C along with foods high in iron to improve the absorption of iron. For instance, a lentil and spinach salad with a side of citrus fruits can be both nutritious and delicious.

4. Mindful Snacking:

Choose nutrient-dense snacks such as nuts, seeds, and fruits. These snacks can provide essential vitamins and minerals while keeping energy levels stable.

5. Hydration is Key:

Ensure you stay well-hydrated. Water helps in nutrient transport and can aid in digestion. Flavor can be added to water and herbal teas without gaining extra calories.

6. Supplements:

Consult with your healthcare provider to determine if supplements are necessary. Vitamin B12, iron, and omega-3 fatty acids are commonly supplemented in vegetarian and vegan pregnancies.

7. Listen to Your Body:

Pay attention to your body's signals. If cravings lead you to specific nutrient-rich foods, indulge sensibly. Cravings are often your body's way of signaling nutritional needs.

8. Meal Planning:

Plan your meals ahead to ensure a balanced intake. Include a variety of vegetables, fruits, whole grains, and plant-based proteins in your daily diet.

9. Educate Yourself:

Stay informed about the nutritional content of foods and explore new recipes. A diverse diet is not only nutritionally sound but also keeps your taste buds engaged.

10. Regular Check-Ups:

Schedule regular check-ups with your healthcare provider. They can monitor your nutritional status and offer guidance based on your specific needs.

In conclusion, a well-balanced vegetarian or vegan pregnancy diet is entirely achievable with thoughtful planning. By embracing a variety of plant-based foods and supplementing wisely, you can ensure both your health and the health of your growing baby. Always consult with your healthcare provider to tailor your diet to your unique needs, making this journey as smooth and joyous as possible.

GLUTEN -FREE OPTIONS

Living a gluten-free lifestyle doesn't mean sacrificing flavor or variety in your diet. Whether you have celiac disease or gluten sensitivity, navigating the world of gluten-free options can be both delicious and satisfying with the right choices.

Understanding Gluten:

Proteins called gluten are present in wheat, barley, rye, and their byproducts. For those with gluten-related disorders, avoiding gluten-containing foods is essential to maintaining good health. Fortunately, there's a growing array of gluten-free alternatives available.

Gluten-Free Grains:

1. Quinoa:
   A versatile and nutrient-packed grain, quinoa is an excellent alternative to wheat. Use it as a side dish, as a basis for salads, or in stir-fries.

2. Rice:
   Naturally gluten-free, rice is a staple that can be enjoyed in various forms - brown rice, white rice, or specialty varieties like jasmine or basmati.

3. Corn:

Corn and corn-based products, such as cornmeal and polenta, are naturally gluten-free. These work well in savory as well as sweet recipes.

4. Buckwheat:

Despite its name, buckwheat is unrelated to wheat and is a gluten-free grain. Buckwheat flour is an excellent choice for pancakes, crepes, and even some types of noodles.

Gluten-Free Flours:

1. Almond Flour:

Almond flour, made from finely ground almonds, adds a delightful nutty flavor to baked goods. It's high in protein and healthy fats.

2. Coconut Flour:

Rich in fiber and low in carbohydrates, coconut flour is an excellent gluten-free alternative. It absorbs a lot of liquid, so recipes may need adjustment.

3. Oat Flour:

Although oats don't contain gluten by nature, cross-contamination can happen when processing them. Look for certified gluten-free oats or oat flour for a safe option.

4. Chickpea Flour:

Also known as gram flour or besan, chickpea flour is a protein-packed option for both savory and sweet dishes.

Navigating Gluten-Free Meals:

1. Fresh Fruits and Vegetables:

Naturally gluten-free, fruits and vegetables are the foundation of a healthy gluten-free diet. Incorporate a colorful variety to ensure a range of nutrients.

2. Proteins:

Focus on lean proteins like poultry, fish, eggs, and legumes. These options provide essential nutrients without the worry of gluten.

3. Dairy:

Most dairy products are gluten-free, but it's essential to be cautious with flavored or processed varieties. Plain milk, yogurt, and cheese are safe choices.

4. Gluten-Free Labels:

When shopping for packaged foods, look for products labeled as gluten-free. It ensures that the item is free from gluten or contains a negligible amount.

Eating Out Gluten-Free:

1. Communication is Key:
Notify the restaurant personnel of your dietary requirements when you are dining out. Many places are accommodating and can suggest gluten-free alternatives.

2. Explore International Cuisine:
Ethnic cuisines like Mexican, Thai, or Japanese often offer gluten-free options. Explore these menus for a variety of flavorful choices.

3. Be Cautious with Sauces:
Gluten can hide in sauces and dressings. Ask for these on the side or inquire about gluten-free alternatives.

Gluten-Free Snacking:

1. Nuts and Seeds:
Snack on a handful of nuts or seeds for a satisfying crunch. They're a great source of healthy fats and protein.

2. Popcorn:

Air-popped popcorn is a wholesome gluten-free snack. Try varying the seasonings to add more taste.

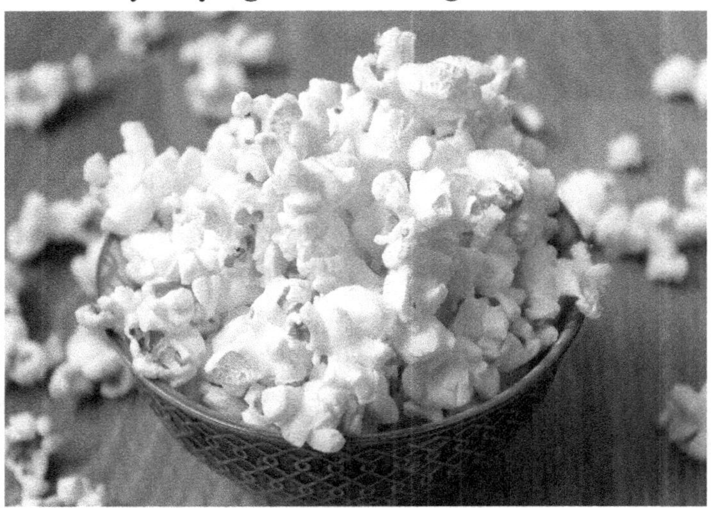

3. Fruit and Cheese:

Pairing fresh fruit with cheese is a delightful and gluten-free combination.

Final Thoughts:

Releasing gluten doesn't have to mean compromising on flavor or variety. With the abundance of gluten-free grains, flours, and fresh ingredients available, you can create a diverse and satisfying menu. Whether cooking at home or dining out, being mindful of your choices and exploring new options can make the gluten-free journey both enjoyable and health-conscious.

MANAGING GESTATIONAL DIABETES THROUGH DIET

Gestational diabetes, a condition that develops during pregnancy, requires careful attention to diet to ensure both the mother's and baby's well-being. Managing gestational diabetes through a balanced and thoughtful diet can help regulate blood sugar levels and reduce the risk of complications. In this chapter, we'll provide practical tips that are easy to incorporate into your daily routine.

Understanding Gestational Diabetes

Gestational diabetes occurs when the body cannot produce enough insulin to meet the increased needs during pregnancy. This leads to elevated blood sugar levels, which, if not managed, can pose risks for both the mother and the baby. The good news is that with proper dietary adjustments, the condition can often be effectively managed.

Balanced Meals and Snacks

Start by focusing on balanced meals and snacks throughout the day. Include a variety of nutrient-rich foods such as whole grains, lean proteins, fruits, and vegetables. Opt for complex carbohydrates like brown rice and whole wheat bread, which are absorbed more slowly, helping to control blood sugar levels.

Mindful Portion Control

Take note of serving quantities to prevent blood sugar increases. Use smaller plates to naturally limit portion sizes and consider dividing your plate into sections – one-half for vegetables, one-fourth for protein, and one-fourth for carbohydrates. This simple approach can help you maintain a balanced intake.

Choose Healthy Fats

Consume foods high in healthful fats, such as almonds, avocados, and olive oil. These fats can help stabilize blood sugar levels and provide essential nutrients. Limit saturated and trans fats found in fried foods and processed snacks, as they can contribute to insulin resistance.

Spread Out Carbohydrate Intake

Rather than consuming large amounts of carbohydrates in one sitting, spread your intake throughout the day.This can stop blood sugar levels from rising suddenly. Choose complex carbohydrates, and pair them with protein and fiber to slow down digestion and absorption.

Regular Meal Timing

Establish a consistent eating schedule. Aim for three balanced meals and two to three snacks each day, spacing them evenly. This routine can help regulate blood sugar levels and provide a steady source of energy.

Stay Hydrated

Water is essential for everyone, especially for those with gestational diabetes.Both blood sugar regulation and general health are supported by it. Drink less sugary beverages and more water or herbal teas.

Monitor Blood Sugar Levels

Regularly monitor your blood sugar levels as advised by your healthcare provider. This will help you understand how different foods affect your body and enable you to make informed choices about your diet.

Collaborate with a Registered Dietitian

Working with a registered dietitian specializing in gestational diabetes can provide personalized guidance. They can help you create a customized meal plan and offer ongoing support and education.

Conclusion

Managing gestational diabetes through diet involves making thoughtful choices to support optimal health for both you and your baby. By adopting these practical tips, you can take control of your nutrition, regulate blood sugar levels, and enjoy a healthy pregnancy. Remember, small changes can make a significant difference, and your healthcare team is there to support you every step of the way.

CHAPTER 8:
CREATING A HEALTHY ENVIRONMENT

In the pursuit of a healthier lifestyle, the environment we surround ourselves with plays a pivotal role. Let me share my personal journey and the transformative power of creating a healthy environment.

Embracing Change

Creating a healthy environment starts with acknowledging the need for change. I found that small, intentional modifications can lead to significant improvements in overall well-being. Begin by evaluating your surroundings—home, workplace, and daily routines.

The Home Oasis

Your home should be a sanctuary that fosters well-being. Simple adjustments, like decluttering, can make a substantial impact. A tidy space reduces stress and promotes a sense of calm. Introduce elements of nature, such as indoor plants, to enhance air quality and add a touch of serenity.

In my own experience, I transformed my kitchen into a hub for nutritious choices. Stocking up on fresh fruits, vegetables, and whole grains makes it easier to opt for wholesome meals. Displaying these items prominently encourages better eating habits for everyone in the household.

Mindful Workspaces

For those of us spending a significant portion of our day at work, crafting a healthy environment in the office is crucial. Incorporate ergonomic furniture, introduce natural light, and take short breaks for stretching exercises. These adjustments not only improve physical health but also boost productivity and focus.

Rituals of Wellness

Establishing daily rituals can be a game-changer. From morning stretches to evening walks, these rituals anchor a healthy routine. I discovered the rejuvenating power of a morning routine that includes meditation and a nutritious breakfast. It sets a positive tone for the day and enhances mental clarity.

Social Connections

Healthy environments extend beyond physical spaces; they encompass social connections. Develop connections with people who inspire and encourage you. Surround yourself with a support system that encourages your well-being journey. Shared experiences and motivations create a reinforcing loop of positivity.

The Technology Balance

In today's digital age, managing screen time is essential for mental and emotional health. Establish boundaries for device usage, especially before bedtime. Creating a tech-free zone in communal areas of your home fosters better interpersonal connections and quality sleep.

Sustainable Living

A healthy environment also involves being mindful of our impact on the planet. Adopting sustainable practices, such as reducing single-use plastics and conserving energy, not only benefits the environment but also contributes to a sense of global well-being.

Conclusion

In conclusion, the power to create a healthy environment lies within our daily choices and intentional actions. By making gradual adjustments, I witnessed a remarkable transformation in my overall well-being. Embrace change, personalize your spaces, foster positive relationships, and prioritize your mental and physical health. Your environment can be a source of inspiration and support on your journey to a healthier, happier life.

TIPS FOR SMART GROCERY SHOPPING

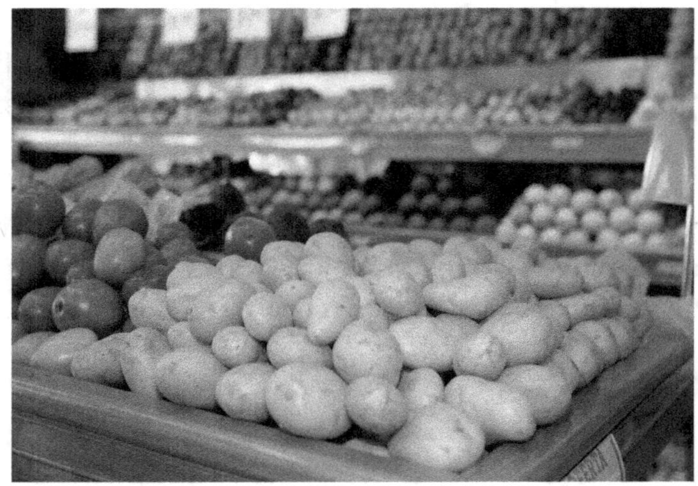

Smart grocery shopping is a key aspect of maintaining a healthy and balanced diet, especially when managing conditions like gestational diabetes. By making informed choices at the grocery store, you can set the foundation for better blood sugar control and overall well-being. Here are some practical tips to make your grocery shopping experience both efficient and health-conscious.

1. Plan Ahead:

Before hitting the grocery store, take a moment to plan your meals for the week. Create a list of essential items, including fresh produce, lean proteins, whole grains, and healthy snacks. Planning helps you stay focused and avoids impulse purchases that may not align with your dietary goals.

2. Shop the Perimeter:

The outer aisles of the grocery store typically house fresh produce, dairy, and protein sources. These areas are your go-to for nutrient-dense foods. Load up on colorful fruits and vegetables, lean meats, and low-fat dairy products to create a well-balanced and diabetes-friendly diet.

3. Read Labels Carefully:

Pay close attention to food labels, especially when choosing packaged items. Look for products with low added sugars and minimal processing. Check the serving size, total carbohydrates, and fiber content to make informed decisions that align with your dietary needs.

4. Choose Whole Grains:

Refined grains should be avoided in favor of whole grains like quinoa, brown rice, and whole wheat bread. Whole grains provide essential nutrients and fiber, promoting better blood sugar control. Be mindful of portion sizes to manage your carbohydrate intake effectively.

5. Prioritize Lean Proteins:

Include lean protein sources such as poultry, fish, tofu, and legumes in your shopping cart. These proteins can help regulate blood sugar levels and provide essential nutrients without excess saturated fats.

6. Stock Up on Healthy Snacks:

Keep your kitchen well-stocked with nutritious snacks to curb cravings and prevent unhealthy choices. Nuts, seeds, Greek yogurt, and fresh fruit make excellent options for satisfying your hunger between meals.

7. Limit Processed Foods:

Minimize your intake of processed and pre-packaged foods, as they often contain hidden sugars, unhealthy fats, and excess sodium. Stick to whole, unprocessed foods to ensure you're nourishing your body with quality nutrients.

8. Stay Hydrated:

Don't forget to include water on your shopping list. It's important to stay hydrated for general health and to help manage appetite.Consider carrying a reusable water bottle to encourage regular water intake throughout the day.

9. Be Mindful of Portions:

While shopping, be mindful of portion sizes to avoid overeating. Choose smaller packaging for snacks or consider dividing larger quantities into smaller portions at home to prevent unintentional overconsumption.

10. Take Advantage of Sales and Discounts:

Explore for offers and savings on nutritious food products. Buying in bulk when items are on sale can save you money in the long run and ensure you always have nutritious options at hand.

By incorporating these practical tips into your grocery shopping routine, you can make informed choices that support your gestational diabetes management goals. Remember, a well-planned and health-conscious shopping trip is a positive step towards maintaining a balanced and nourishing diet.

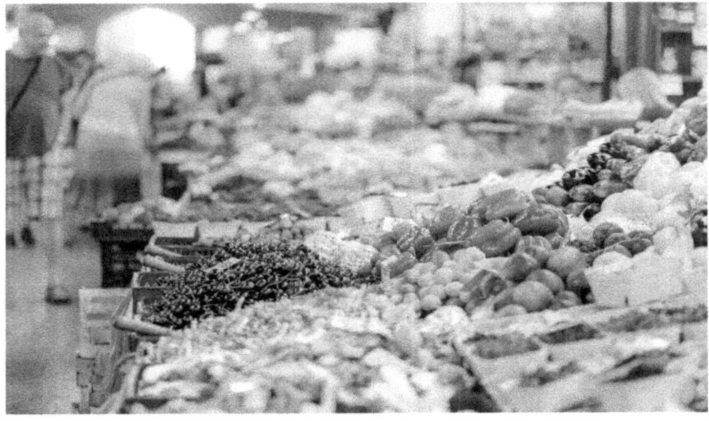

MEAL PLANNING FOR PREGNANCY

It's an amazing adventure once you're pregnant, and eating well is essential to maintaining your health and the wellbeing of your unborn child. Meal planning during pregnancy ensures you get the right mix of nutrients essential for this special time. Here are some practical tips to guide you in crafting nutritious and satisfying meals throughout your pregnancy.

1. Variety is Key:

Try to fill your plate with as many different kinds of fruits and vegetables as possible. Different colors often signify diverse nutrients, and this variety helps cover a broad spectrum of vitamins and minerals essential for fetal development.

2. Balanced Nutrients:

Make sure the macronutrients—proteins, healthy fats, and carbohydrates—are balanced in your meals. Carbohydrates provide energy, proteins support tissue development, and healthy fats are crucial for brain and organ development.

3. Folate-Rich Foods:

Folate is vital during the early stages of pregnancy for preventing neural tube defects. Include foods like leafy greens, legumes, and fortified cereals to meet your folate requirements.

4. Calcium Sources:

Calcium is essential for bone development in your baby. Incorporate dairy products, fortified plant-based milk, and leafy greens into your meals to ensure you're getting an adequate amount of calcium.

5. Iron-Rich Foods:

Iron helps prevent anemia and supports the increased blood volume during pregnancy. Include lean meats, beans, lentils, and fortified cereals to boost your iron intake.

6. Hydration is Key:

Staying hydrated is crucial for both you and your baby. Aim for at least eight 8-ounce glasses of water per day, and consider incorporating hydrating foods like water-rich fruits and vegetables into your meals.

7. Smaller, Frequent Meals:

To ease digestion and manage nausea, consider having smaller, more frequent meals throughout the day. This approach helps regulate blood sugar levels and provides a steady supply of nutrients.

8. Limit Caffeine and Avoid Harmful Foods:
While a moderate amount of caffeine is generally considered safe, it's wise to limit intake during pregnancy. Additionally, steer clear of raw seafood, undercooked meats, and unpasteurized dairy products to minimize the risk of foodborne illnesses.

9. Smart Snacking:
Keep nutritious snacks on hand for those moments between meals. Nuts, yogurt, fruits, and whole-grain crackers make excellent choices to satisfy cravings while providing essential nutrients.

10. Listen to Your Body:
Be mindful of your body's cues and desires. If you're experiencing specific cravings, try to find healthy alternatives that still satisfy your taste buds while meeting your nutritional needs.

11. Consult Your Healthcare Provider:
Each pregnancy is different, and so are the dietary requirements of each individual. Regularly consult with your healthcare provider to ensure you're meeting your specific dietary requirements and to address any concerns or questions you may have.

Meal planning during pregnancy is about nourishing both yourself and your growing baby. By adopting a balanced and varied approach, you can create meals that not only support optimal fetal development but also keep you feeling energized and well-nourished throughout this extraordinary journey.

Making Nutrient-Dense Choices

In the maze of food options available, making nutrient-dense choices is like giving your body a VIP pass to optimal health. Nutrient density is all about getting the most bang for your nutritional buck – choosing foods packed with essential vitamins, minerals, and other vital nutrients without unnecessary calories. Let's dive into practical tips on how you can make nutrient-dense choices a cornerstone of your daily eating habits.

1. Focus on Whole Foods:
   The foundation of nutrient-dense eating is whole foods. These are minimally processed foods that are as near to their natural state as possible. Think of fresh fruits, vegetables, lean proteins, whole grains, and nuts. They come loaded with nutrients in a package your body readily recognizes and utilizes.

2. Color Your Plate:
   Imagine your plate as a canvas, and the more colors you add, the more nutrients you're likely to get. Different colors often signify different nutrients. Aim for a vibrant mix of greens, reds, oranges, and yellows on your plate. Each hue brings a unique set of benefits, contributing to a well-rounded and nutrient-packed meal.

3. Prioritize Leafy Greens:

When it comes to nutrient density, leafy greens are superheroes. Spinach, kale, Swiss chard, and collard greens are bursting with vitamins A, C, K, and folate. They're also rich in minerals like iron and calcium. Sneak them into salads, smoothies, or sautés for a nutrient boost.

4. Opt for Lean Proteins:

Protein is essential for immunological response, muscle regeneration, and general bodily upkeep. Choose lean protein sources like poultry, fish, tofu, legumes, and low-fat dairy products. These options provide the protein punch without excessive saturated fats often found in fattier cuts of meat.

5. Embrace Whole Grains:

Swap refined grains for whole grains to level up your nutrient intake. Whole grains like quinoa, brown rice, oats, and whole wheat contain fiber, B-vitamins, and minerals. They provide sustained energy and contribute to a healthy digestive system.

6. Snack Smart:

Snacking can be a nutrient-dense affair too. Instead of reaching for empty-calorie snacks, opt for nutrient-rich options. Grab a handful of nuts for healthy fats, a piece of fruit for vitamins, or Greek yogurt for protein. These snacks keep you fueled and provide valuable nutrients.

7. Read Labels with Care:
Not all packaged foods are created equal. When choosing packaged items, read labels carefully. Look for foods with short ingredient lists, recognizable components, and minimal additives. Pay attention to serving sizes and the nutritional content per serving.

8. Choose Healthy Fats:
Not all fats are the enemy. Choose healthy fat sources such as nuts, olive oil, avocados, and fatty seafood. These fats are rich in omega-3 fatty acids, which support heart health and provide essential nutrients for overall well-being.

9. Minimize Added Sugars:
Sweet treats can be delightful, but excessive added sugars can detract from nutrient density. Reduce the amount of processed foods, sodas, and sugary snacks you consume. Instead, satisfy your sweet tooth with naturally sweet options like fruits.

10. Stay Hydrated:
Water is the unsung hero of nutrient density. It helps transport nutrients throughout your body, aids

digestion, and keeps your skin glowing. Make water your beverage of choice and limit sugary drinks that can add unnecessary calories without significant nutritional value.

11. Be Mindful of Portions:

While nutrient-dense foods are rich in goodness, portion control still matters. Even nutrient-dense foods contribute calories, and overeating, even on healthy choices, can lead to weight gain. Listen to your body's hunger and fullness cues to maintain a healthy balance.

12. Mix It Up:

Variety is not only the spice of life but also the key to nutrient density. Your body cannot get all the nutrients it needs from a single diet. Mix up your choices to ensure you get a broad spectrum of vitamins, minerals, and other essential nutrients.

In Conclusion:

Making nutrient-dense choices doesn't require a degree in nutrition or a complete overhaul of your eating habits. It's about making small, intentional changes that add up to a big impact on your health. By focusing on whole foods, embracing a colorful plate, and being mindful of the nutritional content of your choices, you can nourish your body with the nutrients it craves. Remember, it's not about perfection but progress. Making nutrient-dense choices is a journey towards a healthier, happier you.

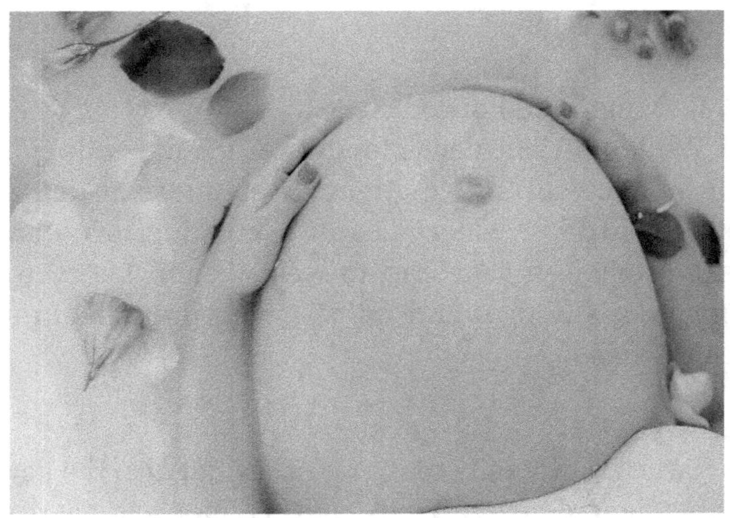

CONCLUSION

Congratulations on completing the chapters of the Pregnancy Diet Cookbook. As we wrap up this journey together, let's reflect on the path you've traversed, understand the lasting impacts of a healthy pregnancy diet, explore the importance of balance beyond pregnancy, discover resources for continued wellness, and celebrate the profound nourishment found in your choices.

Reflecting on Your Pregnancy Journey

Embarking on the remarkable journey of pregnancy is a time filled with emotions, transformations, and, undoubtedly, a multitude of experiences. As you reach the culmination of this beautiful phase, taking a moment to reflect on your pregnancy journey can be a poignant and empowering exercise. Let's explore practical tips to guide you through this reflection, celebrating the unique moments that have shaped this extraordinary chapter in your life.

1. Create a Pregnancy Journal:

Consider starting a pregnancy journal if you haven't already. Documenting your thoughts, feelings, and experiences can provide a tangible record of this incredible journey. Capture the milestones, cravings, and even the challenges you faced. Your journal becomes a personal narrative, a treasure trove of memories to revisit in the years to come.

2. Celebrate Achievements:
Pregnancy is a journey of growth, both for you and your baby. Take a moment to celebrate the achievements, big and small. Whether it's successfully navigating morning sickness or reaching each trimester milestone, acknowledge your resilience and the marvel of creating new life.

3. Embrace Changes:
Your body undergoes remarkable changes during pregnancy. Reflect on how you embraced and adapted to these changes. Appreciate the strength and resilience your body has shown throughout this process. Understanding and accepting the transformations contribute to a positive self-image.

4. Connect with Your Partner:
If you're sharing this journey with a partner, reflect on the ways your relationship evolved during pregnancy. Discuss the challenges you faced together and the moments that strengthened your bond. Open communication about your experiences can deepen your connection.

5. Cherish Ultrasound and Photos:

Your ultrasound images and pregnancy photos capture precious moments in time. Take a moment to reflect on these visual representations of your journey. Consider creating a collage or scrapbook to revisit these images and relive the anticipation and joy they bring.

6. Consider Health and Self-Care:

Reflect on how you prioritized your health and well-being during pregnancy. Consider the self-care practices that brought you comfort, whether it was gentle exercises, prenatal yoga, or moments of relaxation. Recognize the importance of caring for both your physical and emotional health.

7. Connect with Other Moms:

Sharing experiences with fellow moms can be enlightening and comforting. Reflect on the support you received from friends or community groups. Consider continuing these connections post-pregnancy, as the journey of motherhood is one best navigated with a supportive network.

8. Acknowledge Your Emotions:

Pregnancy comes with a rollercoaster of emotions. Take time to acknowledge and reflect on the range of feelings you've experienced – from excitement and joy to anxiety and uncertainty. Understanding these emotions can contribute to a more mindful and positive postpartum experience.

9. Set Realistic Expectations:

Reflect on the expectations you had at the beginning of your pregnancy journey. Assess how these expectations aligned with the reality of your experience. Embrace the unpredictability of parenthood and adjust expectations as needed, fostering a more flexible and adaptive mindset.

10. Plan for Postpartum Support:

As you reflect on your pregnancy journey, start considering the postpartum period. Reflect on the support system you have in place and identify areas where additional assistance may be beneficial. Preparing for the postpartum phase can help ease the transition into the next chapter of your life.

11. Capture Your Reflections:

Take a moment to sit quietly and reflect on your pregnancy journey. Consider writing a letter to yourself, expressing your thoughts, feelings, and hopes for the future. This letter can serve as a beautiful memento and a source of inspiration as you move forward into motherhood.

In Conclusion:

Reflecting on your pregnancy journey is a personal and heartfelt exercise that allows you to honor the incredible transformation you've undergone. Through celebrating achievements, acknowledging changes, and connecting with your emotions, you pave the way for a more conscious and empowered transition into the next chapter. As you embark on the adventure of parenthood, carry the lessons and memories of your pregnancy journey with you, cherishing the uniqueness of this transformative experience.

CELEBRATING THE POWER OF NUTRIENT-RICH FOODS

In the journey towards a healthier and more vibrant life, nutrient-rich foods emerge as unsung heroes, whispering tales of wellness and vitality. Let's celebrate the power of these nutritional powerhouses that not only nourish our bodies but also weave a tapestry of well-being. Here are practical tips to help you revel in the goodness of nutrient-rich foods.

1. Savor the Colors of Nutrition:

Nutrient-rich foods often come in a palette of vibrant colors. Every color represents a different set of nutrients. From the deep greens of leafy vegetables to the rich oranges of sweet potatoes, savor the visual feast of colors on your plate. The more varied the colors, the broader the spectrum of nutrients you're likely consuming.

2. Make Every Bite Count:

Eating nutrient-rich foods isn't just about filling your stomach; it's about fueling your body with essential nutrients. With each bite, appreciate the vitamins, minerals, and antioxidants that contribute to your overall health. Make every meal a conscious act of nourishment.

3. Embrace Whole Foods:

The magic of nutrient density often resides in whole foods. Whole grains, fruits, vegetables, lean proteins, and nuts carry an abundance of nutrients in their unprocessed form. Embrace the simplicity and purity of whole foods to maximize their nutritional benefits.

4. Share the Joy of Nutrient-Rich Meals:

Celebrate the power of nutrient-rich foods by sharing delicious, healthful meals with loved ones. Gather around the table, savoring the flavors of nutrient-dense dishes together. The joy of good food is even more delightful when shared.

5. Explore Culinary Creativity:

Nutrient-rich foods invite culinary creativity. Experiment with new recipes that incorporate a variety of nutrient-dense ingredients. From creating colorful salads to crafting nourishing smoothie bowls, let your kitchen become a canvas for nutritious culinary artistry.

6. Educate Yourself:

Understanding the nutritional value of foods empowers you to make informed choices. Educate yourself about the nutrients present in different foods and their benefits. Knowledge is the key to making mindful decisions that align with your health goals.

7. Keep Hydration in Mind:
Celebrating nutrient-rich foods goes hand in hand with staying hydrated. Digestion, vitamin absorption, and general health all depend on water. Pair nutrient-dense meals with a refreshing glass of water to enhance the benefits of your culinary choices.

8. Make Healthy Swaps:
Infuse your daily meals with nutrient-rich alternatives. Swap refined grains for whole grains, opt for lean proteins, and choose healthy fats. These simple swaps contribute to a diet rich in essential nutrients while still allowing you to enjoy delicious and satisfying meals.

9. Revel in Seasonal Delights:
Nutrient-rich foods often follow the rhythm of the seasons. Celebrate the goodness of seasonal fruits and vegetables, relishing the flavors that nature offers at different times of the year. Seasonal eating not only provides variety but also aligns with your body's natural needs.

10. Express Gratitude for Well-Being:
Take a moment to express gratitude for the well-being that nutrient-rich foods bring to your life. Acknowledge the positive impact on your energy levels, mood, and overall health. Gratitude enhances the joy of nourishing your body with foods that support your vitality.

In Conclusion:
Celebrating the power of nutrient-rich foods is a journey of embracing delicious, wholesome choices that fuel your body and spirit. With an appreciation for the colors, flavors, and nourishment these foods bring, you embark on a path of wellness. Through culinary creativity, mindful choices, and a gratitude-filled approach, savor the journey of nurturing your body with the bountiful power of nutrient-rich foods.

CONTINUING A HEALTHY LIFESTYLE BEYOND PREGNANCY

As the journey of pregnancy unfolds into the realm of motherhood, the echoes of a healthy lifestyle continue to resonate. The habits formed during pregnancy are not just for a season; they're the foundation for a lifetime of well-being for both you and your little one. Let's explore practical tips for seamlessly transitioning into and continuing a healthy lifestyle beyond pregnancy.

1. Embrace Postpartum Self-Care:
Postpartum self-care is a continuation of the nurturing practices initiated during pregnancy. Take time for yourself, prioritize rest, and maintain the habits that contribute to your physical and emotional well-being. A healthy, cared-for mother lays the groundwork for a thriving family.

2. Include the Whole Family:
A healthy lifestyle is a family affair. Involve your partner and other family members in your wellness journey. Plan nutritious meals together, engage in physical activities as a family, and create a

supportive environment that fosters health for everyone.

3. Prioritize Nutrient-Rich Foods:
Continue the celebration of nutrient-rich foods that began during pregnancy.Be certain your meals include a range of vibrant fruits, veggies, whole grains, lean meats, and healthy fats. Nutrient-dense foods are the building blocks of a resilient and thriving body.

4. Make Exercise a Family Affair:
Physical activity is not just a solo venture; it's an opportunity for family bonding. Whether it's a walk in the park, a family bike ride, or a dance session in the living room, make exercise enjoyable and inclusive for everyone.

5. Set Realistic Fitness Goals:
Adjust your fitness goals to accommodate the demands of motherhood. Embrace realistic expectations and find joy in activities that fit seamlessly into your new routine. Consistency over intensity is key to sustaining a long-term healthy lifestyle.

6. Stay Hydrated:
Hydration remains a cornerstone of overall health. Maintain the habit of drinking an adequate amount

of water daily. Staying hydrated supports your energy levels, aids in digestion, and contributes to radiant skin, essential for postpartum well-being.

7. Prioritize Sleep:

Sleep is a precious commodity for new parents. Despite the challenges of irregular sleep patterns with a newborn, prioritize rest as much as possible. Create a sleep-friendly environment and establish bedtime rituals to enhance the quality of your sleep.

8. Foster Mental Well-Being:

Nurturing your mental health is a vital component of a healthy lifestyle. Seek moments of mindfulness, practice gratitude, and be open about your feelings. If needed, don't hesitate to reach out for support from friends, family, or professionals.

9. Schedule Regular Check-Ups:

Your journey with healthcare doesn't end with childbirth. Schedule regular check-ups for both you and your baby. Stay informed about vaccinations, monitor developmental milestones, and address any health concerns promptly.

10. Be Kind to Yourself:

Motherhood is a transformative experience, and it's okay not to have all the answers. Be kind to yourself as you navigate the challenges and joys of raising a child. Embrace the learning curve, celebrate small victories, and remember that self-compassion is a fundamental part of a healthy lifestyle.

In Conclusion:
Continuing a healthy lifestyle beyond pregnancy is a natural progression, an ongoing commitment to your well-being and that of your family. By integrating these practical tips into your daily life, you not only sustain the positive habits initiated during pregnancy but also create an environment that nurtures a lifetime of health and happiness. Embrace the journey with love, flexibility, and a deep understanding that a healthy lifestyle is not a destination but a fulfilling and evolving way of life.

APPENDICES

Appendix A: Sample Meal Plans

This section provides sample meal plans tailored to various dietary needs, including gestational diabetes management, postpartum nutrition, and family-friendly options. These meal plans aim to guide readers in creating well-balanced and nourishing meals for different stages of pregnancy and postpartum.

Appendix B: Nutritional Information Charts

Included in this appendix are detailed charts outlining the nutritional content of common foods. These charts cover macronutrients, micronutrients, and calorie counts, aiding readers in making informed decisions about their dietary choices. The information is presented in a clear and organized format for easy reference.

Appendix C: Physical Activity Guides

In this section, readers will find practical guides on incorporating physical activity into their routines. Tailored for different fitness levels and postpartum stages, these guides include simple exercises, workout plans, and tips for staying active. The aim is to support readers in maintaining a healthy lifestyle beyond pregnancy.

Appendix D: Grocery Shopping Checklist

A comprehensive grocery shopping checklist is provided, offering readers a handy tool for navigating the aisles with a focus on nutrient-dense foods. This checklist is organized by food categories, helping readers create well-rounded and health-conscious shopping lists for their families.

Appendix E: Recommended Reading List

Curated for further exploration, this list includes recommended books, articles, and websites covering a range of topics related to pregnancy, nutrition, and overall well-being. Readers can use this appendix to delve deeper into specific areas of interest or seek additional information from reliable sources.

Appendix F: Glossary of Terms

For clarity and understanding, a glossary of key terms used throughout the book is provided. This resource ensures that readers can easily reference and comprehend any terminology that may be unfamiliar. Definitions are presented in a concise and reader-friendly format.

Appendix G: Contact Information for Health Professionals

To foster a proactive approach to healthcare, this section includes contact information for various health professionals, such as dietitians, obstetricians, and fitness experts. Readers can use this appendix to connect with professionals who can provide personalized guidance based on their individual needs.

Appendix H: Blank Meal Planning Templates

Encouraging readers to actively engage in their dietary choices, this section includes blank meal planning templates. These templates can be filled in with personal preferences and dietary requirements, serving as practical tools for organizing and customizing meal plans.

Formatting Note: Appendices are listed in alphabetical order for easy navigation. Each appendix is labeled with a clear and concise title. The content within each appendix is presented in a standardized format, making it reader-friendly and conducive to quick reference.